Laboratory Procedures for
Full and Partial Dentures

General Series Editor
J. M. Mumford

Also by the same author
Laboratory Procedures for
Inlays, Crowns and Bridges

Laboratory Procedures for
Full and Partial Dentures

DEREK STANANOUGHT   *FBIST; FRSA*

Senior Lecturer in Dental Technology
John Dalton Faculty of Technology
Manchester Polytechnic

Edited by

A. V. NEWTON   *MDS*

Senior Lecturer in Operative Dental Surgery
University of Liverpool

Consultant in charge of the Prosthetic Department
Liverpool Dental Hospital

Blackwell Scientific Publications
Oxford London Edinburgh Melbourne

© 1978 Blackwell Scientific Publications
Osney Mead, Oxford OX2 0EL
8 John Street, London WC1N 2ES
9 Forrest Road, Edinburgh EH1 2QH
P.O. Box 9, North Balwyn, Victoria, Australia

First published 1978

British Library Cataloguing in Publication Data
Stananought, Derek
    Laboratory procedures for full and partial dentures.
    1. Dentures   2. Dentistry – Laboratory manuals
    I. Title
    617.6'92'028   RK656

    ISBN 0–632–00133–X

Distributed in the U.S.A. by
J. B. Lippincott Company, Philadelphia

and in Canada by
J. B. Lippincott Company of Canada Ltd, Toronto

Phototypeset in V.I.P. Times by
Western Printing Services Ltd, Bristol
Printed and bound in Great Britain by
Billing & Sons Ltd,
Guildford, London and Worcester

Contents

Editor's foreword

This book is the companion volume to *Laboratory Procedures for Inlays, Crowns and Bridges*. It represents an attempt to present to technicians, apprentice technicians, dental students and dentists an integrated, practical approach to modern dental technology. It is essentially a laboratory manual, intended for use at the bench as well as for general reading. The book covers a wide sector of dental technology which excludes only such appliances as precision attachments, maxillofacial splints and the more complicated variants of the metal skeleton denture.

A further aim has been to provide a clear, unambiguous text for student technicians, which will be sufficiently comprehensive to prepare them for national examinations.

A. V. NEWTON

Preface

The aim of this book is to instruct undergraduate clinicians and dental technicians in the procedures involved in constructing full and partial dentures.

A recommended reading list is given in the Appendix which will provide readers with information on the theoretical background to the procedures described and the materials used.

Students are reminded that the procedures described in this book are not the only methods available—many technicians and clinicians modify procedures learnt in training to suit their own particular needs. However, the procedures described have proved consistently successful over many years.

I wish to thank Mr A. V. Newton for his advice and encouragement during the preparation of this book. A special thank you to Mr H. Harcourt, formerly chief examiner in Dental Technology for the City and Guilds of London Institute, and Mr L. B. Ward, Senior Lecturer in charge of Dental Courses, Manchester Polytechnic, for reading the manuscript and offering guidance and advice. I am indebted to Professor C. P. Adams and Messrs John Wright and Sons Limited of Bristol for permission to modify and describe the method for trimming dental casts from 'The Design and Construction of Removable Orthodontic Appliances'. My thanks also to Mr K. Winfield, Dental Technician, University of Liverpool, for his advice and demonstration of the swaging of stainless steel described in Chapter 8 and for reading this area of the manuscript.

DEREK STANANOUGHT

1 Construction of Casts

Most dental technical procedures are carried out on a cast (model) which is a positive likeness of the tooth-bearing and associated areas of the oral cavity. This is obtained by taking an impression (a negative likeness) of those areas, and pouring a suitably strong material into it to form the cast. It is of prime importance that the cast is an accurate duplicate of the mouth. This normally involves a two-impression technique. The first or primary impression is taken in irreversible hydrocolloid (alginate) or impression compound and supported in a stock tray. The second impression may be taken in irreversible hydrocolloid, rubber base, zinc oxide–eugenol paste or plaster of Paris. These impressions are supported in a tray, termed a special tray, which is constructed to fit the preliminary cast of the patient's oral tissues.

Impressions taken in a thermoplastic material such as impression compound, generally displace the oral tissues because pressure is required to seat them. Such an impression is termed mucocompressive. Materials such as hydrocolloid, rubber base and plaster of Paris exhibit good flow properties and, if handled correctly, do not displace the oral tissues. They are therefore called mucostatic impression materials. If muscles of the oral cavity are flexed during impression-taking, a functional impression is formed, which indicates the boundaries of muscular activity. This information is essential when constructing appliances for the mouth.

When the natural dentition is complete it is said to be fully dentate; if some teeth are missing the mouth is referred to as being partially dentate; and a mouth devoid of teeth is termed edentulous. The terms dentate, partially dentate and edentulous are used to describe impressions and casts alike.

1

PRELIMINARY CASTS

Preliminary casts may be used to:

1   Analyse the feasibility of various restorative measures.

2   Analyse the relationship between maxilla and mandible, when the casts are articulated (see Chapter 9).

3   Analyse the static and dynamic relationship of the chewing surfaces of opposing teeth (see occlusion and articulation, Chapter 9).

4   Analyse in the laboratory the details of specified areas of the oral cavity.

5   Make a permanent record of required areas of the oral cavity.

6   Help the dentist to discuss possible forms of treatment with the technician and patient.

7   Provide a foundation for the construction of special trays (see p. 11).

The material in which the cast is to be formed should be compatible with all types of impression material and be easy to use, with a reasonable setting time. It should also reproduce surface detail from the impression, exhibit high surface hardness and strength (sufficient to withstand normal working loads) with no expansion or contraction and be compatible with materials used in the construction of dental appliances from which they should be easily removable.

Derivatives of gypsum called plaster of Paris (β hemihydrate of calcium sulphate) and dental stone (α hemihydrate of calcium sulphate) are used extensively for casts. Dental stone is stronger than plaster of Paris and so is reserved for procedures where strength is essential. Both materials are supplied in powder form, which when added to water is converted to the dihydrate form of calcium sulphate and becomes hard. Their gross physical properties are affected by and controlled by:

1   Powder to water ratio. A high powder to water ratio produces a thick mix which sets quickly, exhibits increased expansion and good surface hardness, but is difficult to pour into an impression. Conversely, a mixture of low powder to water ratio is slow to set, its expansion is low, surface hardness poor but it is comparatively easy to pour. Consequently, a compromise must be achieved which gives reasonable working time and satisfactory physical properties. Powder–water ratios are given in the appropriate sections throughout the book.

2 Spatulation time. This is the time taken to mix the powder and water to a creamy consistency. Normally 30–60 seconds is sufficient to produce a satisfactory mix. A long spatulation time decreases the surface hardness, increases the expansion and produces a rapid set. A short spatulation time has the reverse effect.

3 Temperature of the water. An increase in the water temperature up to a maximum of 40°C decreases the setting time. Water temperature above 40°C increases the setting time of plaster of Paris.

4 Chemical additives. Chemicals such as potassium sulphate and sodium chloride may be used to decrease the setting time, whilst borax is used to increase it.

Precautions should be taken to prevent impressions being distorted in the interval before casts are poured. The surface of the impression must not be submitted to pressure, therefore the tray should be supported in such a way that the posterior border does not make contact with, for example, a bench top. Hydrocolloid impression materials should be prevented from losing or gaining water. Water tends to evaporate from a colloidal gel, which results in the more soluble constituents of the hydrocolloid exuding on to its surface. The exudate can effect the setting of calcium sulphate on contact. Evaporation and absorption of water produces a distortion of the impression material. Therefore, the impression should be placed in a self-seal plastic bag which acts as a humidor, and so prevents a change in the moisture content.

The preliminary cast is poured in the following manner.

1 The impression is washed under cold running water to remove traces of blood or mucus from its surface, and dried by compressed air or with a piece of dental gauze.

2 The impression is placed on a bench designated for plaster-work (termed the plaster bench) in such a manner that the posterior border does not contact the bench. This prevents distortion of the impression and normally results in the tray being parallel to the bench, which is ideal for a later procedure (Fig. 1.1).

3   The cast may be poured in plaster of Paris only, a 50/50 mix of plaster of Paris and a dental stone, such as Kaffir 'D', or in a dental stone only with a base of plaster of Paris. The last method will be described.

Water is poured into a calibrated cylinder, 35 cm³ measured and poured into a clean rubber mixing vessel called a plaster bowl. Dental stone is weighed, 100 g is sufficient for the above amount of water, and sifted slowly into the water. Gentle taps on the side of the bowl help to settle the powder in the water and reduce air inclusions. The contents of the bowl may be mixed either by use of a mechanical spatulator which consists of a geared paddle rotated by a handle, or by use of a hand held spatula which has a curved blade. The slurry of dental stone is pressed against the side of the bowl to remove lumps and so produce a creamy mix. If, during spatulation, the bowl is submitted to a series of rapid taps (vibrated) air inclusions will be liberated from the mix to produce an air-free creamy mix. Vibrations may be introduced by an electrical machine called a vibrator, the bowl being placed on a rubber mat over the vibrating surface.

4   The plaster bowl is removed from the vibrator and placed in a convenient position for the next stage. By taking hold of the handle of the impression tray in one hand and placing the centre of the tray against the edge of the vibrator, small increments of dental stone may be introduced into the impression from the posterior region. A hand held spatula is used for this purpose. Care is taken to vibrate the stone along the floor of the impression slowly, to minimize air inclusions. Vibrations are continued until the impression has been filled to its periphery, when it is again placed with the tray parallel to the bench. More stone is added to a height of 5 mm above the highest part of the impression. Rough protrusions of stone are positioned at random over the exposed surface of the cast (Fig. 1.1). The protrusions are used to bond the cast to a base of plaster of Paris at a later stage. The vibrator is switched off and the stone allowed to set for a minimum of 30 minutes.

5   The plaster bowl and spatula are cleaned under running water.

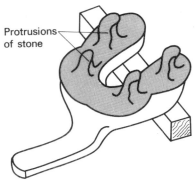

Protrusions of stone

Fig. 1.1   Rough protrusions of dental stone are placed at random over the surface of the cast. The impression is placed with its posterior region supported off the bench.

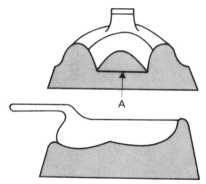

Fig. 1.2 The base of a cast should have an outward taper and the upper surface of the tray should be parallel to the bench. The plaster occupying the lingual aspect of a lower is removed to the edge of the tray (A).

Remnants of set calcium sulphate left on a plaster bowl or spatula will become incorporated in a subsequent dental stone–water mixture and cause it to set quicker.

6 Once the cast of dental stone has set, a base is formed to it (Fig. 1.2), the process is termed basing off. The cast is soaked in cold water for a few minutes to prevent absorption of water from the basing off plaster, which would impair the bond between the two. Plaster of Paris is added to clean water in the ratio of 100 g/50 cm³ and spatulated to a creamy consistency. The cast is removed from the water, and excess water shaken off its surface. The plaster is vibrated over the exposed surface of the cast until the protrusions have been covered. A suitable flexible pad (such as a smooth rubber mat) is placed on the plaster bench and the remainder of plaster placed in a mound on it. Alternatively, a plastic or rubber base former may be filled with the plaster. The cast is inverted into the plaster in such a way that the tray is parallel with the bench, there is a 20 mm thickness of plaster beneath the cast, the plaster extends 5 mm beyond the periphery of the impression and the walls of the base have an outward taper (Fig. 1.2). Plaster of Paris occupying the space between the arms of a lower tray (the lingual aspect) is removed whilst soft until level with the top edge of the impression material (Fig. 1.2). A plaster spatula is used to scrape it away.

7 The plaster is left to set for 1 hour before attempting to remove the impression.

Removal of the impression

The method used to remove an impression material from a cast varies slightly depending upon the material used.

Impression compound

1 Set calcium sulphate and impression compound are removed from the outer surface of the tray by use of a special knife called a plaster knife.

2 The cast is held firmly in one hand with the fingers supporting the tray, and the thumb on the base of the cast. A sharp tap on the handle of the tray with the handle of a plaster knife should release the tray from the impression. If the tray is not removed easily, the following stage should be carried out with the tray attached to the impression. Further tapping is not encouraged because of the possibility of damage to the cast.

3 A plastic or metal bowl is filled with warm water, the temperature of which should be 60°C, and the cast placed in it. Warm water softens the impression compound which allows the tray to be removed. As the compound softens further, it is peeled off the cast by commencing at the posterior border of the impression. Portions firmly adhering to the cast are removed by pressing a ball of softened compound on to the area and then removing it. This softens the adhering portion and lifts it off the cast. The temperature of the water is important; cool water will not soften the compound and very hot water makes the compound sticky and difficult to remove from the cast.

Irreversible hydrocolloid

Excess plaster and stone is removed from the tray; the handle is firmly held in one hand, the cast in the other, and the tray pulled in a vertical direction. Rocking of the tray may fracture the cast. Occasionally, the tray may pull away from the impression material, in which case the impression is gently peeled off the buccal (outer) area of the cast, commencing at its posterior border, and then peeled off the lingual (inner) surface.

Trimming casts

The shape of a cast is important. It must be an accurate reproduction of the mouth with no areas missing and yet be small enough for convenient handling. The procedure of shaping is called trimming and is normally carried out on a mechanical device consisting of an electrical motor to which a large carborundum wheel encased in a metal housing is attached. There is an opening in the housing to which a platform is attached. The cast is placed on the platform and moved through the opening in the housing against the wheel. The wheel is lubricated with water which disposes of the removed calcium sulphate.

Edentulous casts

1 The posterior surface of the cast is straightened by standing its base on the platform of the trimmer and gently pressing the cast against the rotating wheel. It is essential to stop the trimming about 8 mm from the tuberosities or retromolar pads.

2 The cast is placed upright on its posterior surface and the base trimmed so that the edentulous ridge lies approximately in the same plane as it would in the mouth (Fig. 1.3). The base of the cast should be at least 10 mm thick to produce adequate strength.

3 The outer surface of an edentulous cast is trimmed by placing its base on the platform and the sides trimmed to the curvature of the sulcus but about 3 mm from its maximum convexity (Fig. 1.3). The posterior surface of the cast is retrimmed to within 5 mm of the tuberosity or retromolar pad (Fig. 1.3). The finished shape of the

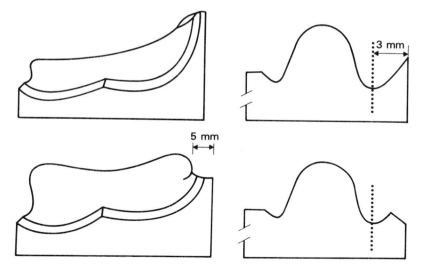

Fig. 1.3 The base of the cast is trimmed so that the edentulous ridge lies approximately in the same plane as it would in the mouth. The sides of the cast are trimmed to within 3 mm of the maximum convexity of the sulcus and the sharp corner produced chamfered away.

cast should be symmetrical when viewed from the reverse side of the base. A sharp corner will be present where the sides of the cast meet the ascending walls of the sulcus. This is removed by a knife to form a 45° angle chamfer about $1\frac{1}{2}$ mm wide (Fig. 1.3).

4   Excess plaster on the lingual aspect of a lower is removed to leave a lingual sulcus approximately 2 mm deep. A flat-bladed sculptor or plaster knife is used (Fig. 1.4). The blade of a sculptor should be short enough to allow the handle to be placed in the palm of the hand with the thumb resting on the side of the cast (Fig. 1.4). Pressure from the hand pushes the sculptor forward but by keeping the thumb rigid prevents more than about 10 mm forward movement. The supporting hand must be kept well clear of the sculptor blade and care taken not to damage the cast.

Partially dentate casts

Partially dentate casts may be trimmed in the manner described for edentulous casts. Alternatively, they may be trimmed in the manner of fully dentate casts described below. This may necessitate the relationship of the mandible to the maxilla being recorded by use of a wax wafer registration (see Chapter 3).

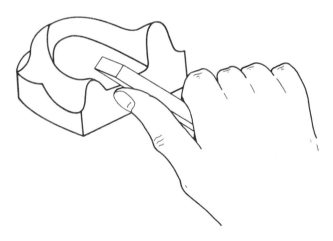

Fig. 1.4   Plaster on the lingual aspect of a lower cast is removed by use of a flat-bladed sculptor.

Fully dentate casts

The base of a fully dentate cast is trimmed with the walls of the upper cast parallel to the walls of the lower cast. This enables the teeth to be accurately occluded with ease (brought together in the manner of clenching the teeth in the mouth) so that the occlusion may be studied.

1   After removal of the impression material, the lower cast is inverted and the occlusal surface of the teeth placed on a block of wood, approximately 8 cm high by 30 cm square. The heels and last molar of the cast should overhang the edge of the block to align the teeth as near as possible to the natural occlusal plane (see Chapter 3). The pointer of an engineer's scribing block is set at one and a half times the anatomical height of the cast (from the sulcus to the occlusal surface of the teeth, Fig. 1.5), placed on the block of wood and used to scribe a line around the base of the cast. The cast is trimmed to this line.

2   The teeth of the upper and lower casts are occluded (Fig. 1.5) and the base of the lower placed on the wood block. The pointer of the scribing block is adjusted to double the previous height and the base of the upper cast scribed and trimmed to the mark (Fig. 1.5).

3   There are many ways of trimming these casts from this stage onwards but a successful method is to use templates in the manner described by Adams (1975, see Appendix). The cast exhibiting the greatest measurement between the canines and between the last molars is the first to be trimmed. Template No. 2 is used to assist with trimming the buccal segments. It is placed on the trimming table of the electric trimmer and the cast moved along its leading edge (Fig. 1.6). The posterior corners are trimmed with the aid of template No. 3 (Fig. 1.6).

4   Upper and lower casts are occluded and the untrimmed cast placed on the trimming table. Trimming is complete when the uppermost cast comes in contact with the cutting wheel. The posterior surfaces of the casts are trimmed simultaneously until 5 mm from the last molar.

5   The anterior region of the casts (that area in the vicinity of the

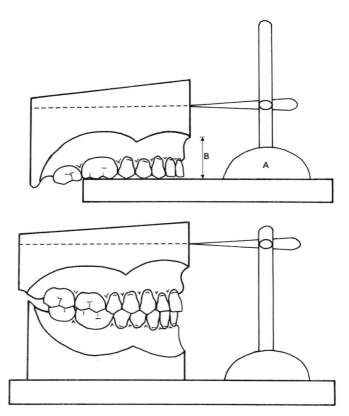

Fig. 1.5 A, an engineer's scribing block is used to define the angle of the base of the cast; B, anatomical height of cast.

front of the mouth) is adjusted separately, uppers being trimmed to a point from the centre of the canines to the centre of the cast ahead of the central teeth (Fig. 1.7). Template No. 1 may be used to produce the required angle (Fig. 1.6). Lowers are given a symmetrical curve from canine to canine, keeping 5 mm from the labial sulcus (Fig. 1.7). Each cast should be symmetrical when viewed from the undersurface.

6 Sharp edges around the sulcus are chamfered. It should be possible to occlude the casts by standing them on their sides on a bench. They may be smoothed with sandpaper and dusted with French chalk to produce a shiny finish.

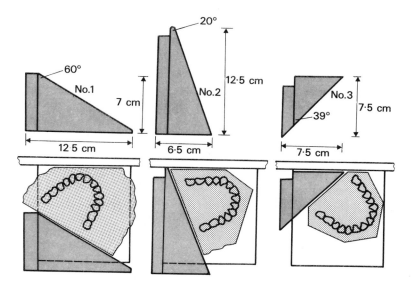

Fig. 1.6 Templates, described by Adams (1975), may be used to assist with the trimming of fully dentate casts.

Laboratory-formed impression trays

Stock impression trays, although convenient are only an approximate fit for any patient's mouth. This results in variations in the thickness of the impression material, localized pressure on the oral tissues, incomplete coverage of the tissues and perhaps distortion of the impression material. Such discrepancies may be overcome by the construction of an accurately fitting tray, called a special tray, made on the preliminary cast. These should be sufficiently strong and rigid not to distort or break whilst in use, be compatible with all impression materials and be relatively cheap and easy to use. Shellac and acrylic resin are materials used for this purpose, shellac being suitable for use with irreversible hydrocolloid and plaster of Paris, whilst acrylic resin, being more rigid, may be used with most known impression materials.

Shellac

Shellac is a thermoplastic material supplied in shapes suitable for upper and lower arch forms. Some materials contain an aluminium

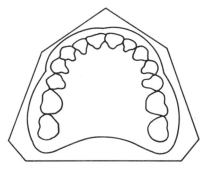

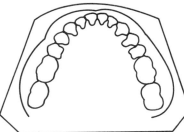

Fig. 1.7 Upper dentate casts are trimmed to a point, whilst the anterior section of lower dentate casts are given a symmetrical curve from canine to canine.

powder which is said to increase the strength and decrease the brittleness of the shellac.

1   Unwanted tooth or tissue undercuts are eliminated on the cast (see Chapter 2).

2   The position of the periphery of the tray is outlined on the cast. It should finish 2 mm short of the sulcus and muscle attachments, to allow for a roll of impression material to record the sulcus.

3   Allowance is made for a 2 mm thickness of impression material by adapting a spacer to the cast. The interstitial spaces between teeth on a partially dentate cast are filled with wax before adapting the spacer. A sheet of modelling wax (approximately 8·0×9·5 cm) is softened above a Bunsen burner flame by moving it to and fro and turning it over at regular intervals to prevent localized melting. The outer edges of the wax are supported whilst the centre is adapted to the palate or lingual aspect of the cast, care being taken to prevent stretching and thinning. If it hardens before adaption is complete, the wax is resoftened and adaption continued. The wax is trimmed to the predetermined outline of the tray by use of a heated wax knife (Fig. 1.8). The spacer is covered with French chalk, followed by one layer of dental napkin to prevent the tray material sticking to the spacer.

4   Shellac is softened over a Bunsen burner flame in the manner described for wax. It is adapted to the palatal or lingual surface of the cast to the crest of the ridge in the edentulous case and to the occlusal surface of the teeth in the partially dentate case. Care is taken to prevent thinning. It is periodically resoftened and the adaptation procedure completed.

5   It is removed from the cast, the edge of the shellac softened and trimmed to a general shape with scissors. After cooling, the tray is held against a bench peg and the periphery of the tray filed to finish at the edge of the wax spacer (Fig. 1.8). It should be noted that shellac is brittle and easily broken during this stage.

6   The tray handle is made from a 20 cm length of 1·5–2·0 mm nickel silver round wire. It is held at its centre in a pair of snipe-nosed pliers and both sides bent in the same direction until they contact at a point 4 cm from the centre of the pliers. Both arms should lie on the same plane. They are bent at 90° and kept in

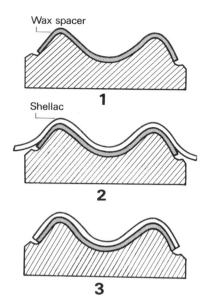

Fig. 1.8 1, a wax spacer is adapted to the cast and trimmed to the predetermined outline of the tray; 2, shellac is softened and adapted over the spacer; 3, the shellac is trimmed to finish at the edge of the wax spacer.

contact for 6 mm then each arm adjusted separately to follow the contour of the dental arch to form retentive arms (Fig. 1.9). The step in the handle allows it to rise over the lip in an edentulous case but a step is not required in a dentate mouth. The handle may be soldered in the area of the step to give strength and rigidity which prevents the handle twisting whilst in use (see Chapter 8 for soldering technique). The handle may be polished (see Chapter 7 for polishing technique).

7 The retentive arms are heated over a Bunsen burner flame and positioned on the tray. The following points are essential:

a The handle should not penetrate the shellac.
b It should have its long axis in line with and directly forward of the midline (centre) of the cast.
c It should be parallel to the base of the cast.
d The step in the handle should lie directly over the centre of the edentulous ridge.

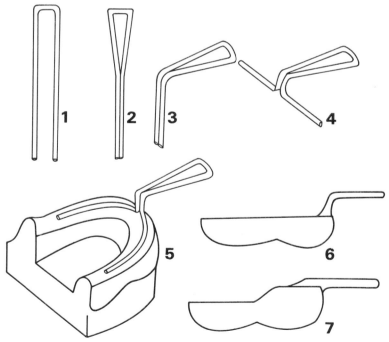

Fig. 1.9 1, 2, 3 and 4, stages in bending a wire handle; 5, the arms are adjusted to follow the contour of the dental arch; 6, side view of a stepped handle; 7, side view of a straight handle used on a special tray for a partially dentate mouth.

Excess shellac removed during the trimming stage of the tray is placed on a wax knife, heated and placed over the retentive arms of the handle. This is repeated until the handle is securely attached to the tray and covered with an even layer of shellac running the whole length of the tray. Careful manipulation of the heated wax knife can produce an initial finish which may be smoothed with a file and sandpaper. Finally, a polish may be obtained by smearing with wax, flaming the surface with a fine Bunsen burner flame, then holding the tray under cold running water and rubbing the waxed surface with wet cotton wool.

8   Irreversible hydrocolloid impressions are difficult to remove from a dentate or partially dentate mouth because the impression material penetrates between the teeth which may result in the tray being pulled off the impression material. Retention, in the form of holes, can be incorporated in a tray by use of a rotating rose-head bur. The holes are drilled about 5 mm apart over the whole of the tray. These allow the impression material to pass through the holes and grip the tray. These trays are called perforated trays and they are given a semi-gloss finish by applying French chalk to the surface of the shellac.

9   The spacer is removed from the cast which is cleaned by pouring boiling water over it. The tray is placed on the cast.

Acrylic resin

Acrylic resin (polymethyl-methacrylate) is supplied in powder–liquid (polymer–monomer) form which when mixed eventually changes into a solid mass. There are many varieties of acrylic resin but they are divided into two specific groups; those requiring heat to harden them and those utilizing a chemical to initiate the hardening process. The hardening process is called polymerization (see Chapter 10) and so they are known respectively as heat-polymerizing (heat cured) and autopolymerizing (cold cured) acrylic resins. Autopolymerizing acrylic resins prepared for the construction of special trays contain a filler to produce a smooth dough. They are more convenient to use than the heat-polymerizing types and so are often used in preference to them. The construction of a special tray using an autopolymerizing acrylic resin is described below.

1   The cast is prepared with a wax spacer into which three small holes, 5 mm × 3 mm, are cut, one in the anterior region of the dental arch and one each in the posterior region. These allow raised portions to be formed on the fitting surface of the tray which act as stops preventing the tray being pressed on to the oral tissues during impression-taking, thereby ensuring an even thickness of material throughout the impression. The spacer is covered with one layer of dental napkin.

2   Monomer (liquid) is poured into a vitreous-surfaced mixing pot and polymer (powder) sifted into it. The proportions vary between manufacturers and their instructions should be followed. The constituents are mixed to a dough consistency and rolled between the fingers into a rod shape. This is flattened into the mould supplied by most manufacturers and laid on a lightly greased surface. Excess material is returned to the mixing pot and covered to prevent evaporation of the monomer.

3   The dough is adapted to the cast rather in the manner of adapting a shellac base plate but without the heating. Care is taken to prevent thinning.

4   A handle, which should be about 15 mm wide, is formed from the excess material in one of two ways; stepped horizontal for normal edentulous ridges, and horizontal for dentate and partially dentate cases (Fig. 1.9). The end of the handle which is to be joined to the tray is moistened with monomer, adapted centrally over the incisal area of the tray and secured with excess acrylic resin which is also moistened with monomer. The handle is supported until polymerization is complete.

5   Shaping is accomplished by trimming on a rotating carborundum wheel mounted on a dental lathe (Fig. 1.10). The tray must not descend below a 45° angle from the centre of the wheel (Fig. 1.10) when it could be pulled beneath the wheel to damage the tray or operator's hands. Final trimming is carried out by use of a rotary instrument (called a rotary trimmer) held in a handpiece. The periphery of the tray should follow the previously determined outline and be smooth with no sharp corners.

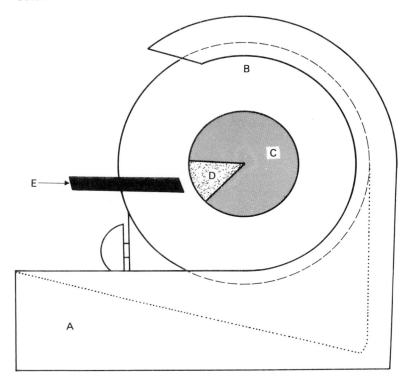

Fig. 1.10 A, rubber trough for confining debris and offering protection to the operator by partially covering the rotating wheel 'C'; B, dental lathe; C, carborundum wheel; D, area of wheel to be used during the grinding operation; E, material being ground.

6 It is smoothed with sandpaper, which may be held in the operator's hand and rubbed across the work or held in a split mandril secured in a handpiece and rotated over the work.

7 The cast is cleaned, and the tray placed on it.

Pressure-formed tray

There are various types of forming apparatus available for compressing a plastic blank to cause it to conform to the shape of a cast. They generally fall into two categories, those using vacuum pressure and those using compressed air. The latter offers greater pressure. The reader is recommended to read the operating instructions for each manufacturer's machine before use. A typical unit may consist of, a table on which the cast is placed, supporting frame for holding the plastic blank, a heating unit for softening the plastic blank, and some means of forming a vacuum or issuing air pressure to the blank. An air pressure method will be described (see Appendix).

1   The cast is placed on the table and the base part of the cast embedded in lead shot. The anatomical section is covered with a piece of 5 mm polyurethane foam which acts as a spacer and simultaneously forms a rough surface to the tray to improve retention of the impression material.

2   The heater is switched on and preheated for about 10 minutes. A plastic blank is clamped in the supporting frame and the heater swivelled over it. Softening occurs from the uppermost surface, penetrating through to the undersurface. Initially, the material appears to rise, then it falls, at which point it is ready for adaptation to the cast. It takes about 2 minutes to reach this stage.

3   Once the blank is soft and pliable, the source of heat is removed, the blank is brought into contact with the cast and air pressure applied. This is normally a simultaneous action. A pressure of approximately 413·7 kN/m² (60 psi) is used for between 1 and 2 minutes.

4   A valve is opened to allow cool air to pass over the plastic sheet and the pressure released. The cast is removed from the table and the shaped blank removed from the cast. Excess tray material is removed by use of an electric cutter or by a bur held in a handpiece. It is finally trimmed with a rotary trimmer.

5   Handles may be purchased, cut from excess plastic blank, or formed in an autopolymerizing acrylic resin. The handle is secured to the tray by a small amount of autopolymerizing acrylic resin. A small amount of resin is mixed to a fluid consistency, placed on the appropriate area of the tray and the handle positioned on the tray. The joint is smoothed by a further addition of acrylic resin, and the handle supported until polymerization is complete. The joint is smoothed by use of a rotary trimmer and sandpaper.

POURING THE MASTER CAST

A cast poured from a second impression is termed a master cast. An accurate impression, devoid of distortion is necessary to produce an accurate duplicate of the mouth. Precautions are taken to prevent pressure on the impression whilst it is being poured by encasing it in a box, this procedure is termed boxing in. The box should be 5 mm larger than the impression to allow for trimming of the cast. It is formed by attaching a roll of wax to the impression tray, just below the periphery of the impression material and attaching a band of stiff material to this to form a box.

1   Carding wax is soft and pliable at room temperature and is ideal when forming the roll to be attached to the tray. The wax is rolled into a 5 mm diameter rod, long enough to encircle the impression tray. It is wrapped around the tray and sealed to it by use of a hot wax knife (Fig. 1.11).

2   The lingual aspect of a lower impression is filled with sheet wax, cut to size and sealed to the wax roll (Fig. 1.11).

3   Sufficient modelling wax, carding wax, waxed bandage, stiff card or thick tin foil is cut to encircle the impression to a height of 4 cm. It is wrapped around the impression and attached to the undersurface of the wax roll by use of further wax. Its walls should be perpendicular or have a slight outward taper with the top edge parallel to the impression tray. Failure to seal the box correctly will result in loss of calcium sulphate from the box during the vibrating stage of pouring the cast. Care must be taken to prevent distortion of the impression material during the formation of the box.

Plaster of Paris impression

If a plaster impression is fractured, as occasionally happens when it is removed from an undercut area in the mouth, the pieces must be accurately repositioned in the tray and sealed to it by an adhesive wax called model cement (sticky wax). Discrepancies are filled with modelling wax. The surface of the impression material is coated with a separating medium to prevent the cast bonding to it. Oil, sodium silicate, proprietary products or soap may be used. Most are painted on and allowed to dry before pouring the cast. Soap is applied on a soft brush (a shaving brush is ideal) to form a lather, which is washed off. This is repeated until a slight sheen is visible on

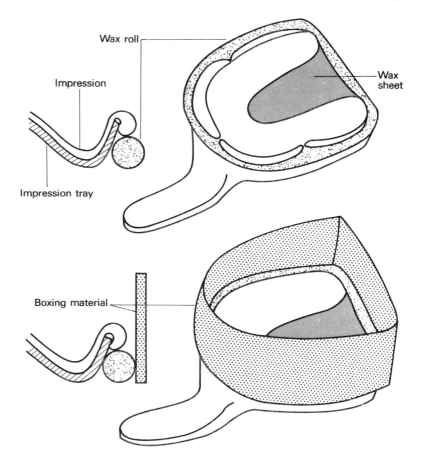

Fig. 1.11 The lingual aspect of a lower impression is filled with sheet wax and a wax roll sealed to the impression tray. Boxing material is attached to the wax roll.

the surface of the impression. Soap forms an insoluble calcium deposit by reaction with the plaster which may result in a roughened surface to the poured cast, unless washed off. The impression material is boxed in.

The cast is poured in dental stone mixed to a powder–water ratio of 100 g/35 cm^3. Small increments of stone are vibrated into the impression until the stone reaches the top of the box. The cast is allowed to harden for 1 hour.

Zinc oxide—eugenol paste impression

This type of impression material may be boxed in the manner described, although it is not absolutely necessary. Zinc oxide–eugenol impression pastes do not require special treatment before pouring the cast.

Hydrocolloids

Hydrocolloids are boxed in the manner described but require no special treatment before pouring the cast.

Elastomers

The rubber base materials are boxed in the manner described. They require no special treatment before pouring a cast but should be dry before doing so.

Removing the impression

The boxed material (wax, tin foil, etc) is removed by breaking its seal with the tray and peeling it off the cast. The tray is then cleaned of stone debris to ensure it is free of the cast.

Plaster impression

1   The cast is held whilst the handle of the tray is tapped to release it from the impression material.
2   Care is taken to prevent damage to the cast during the following procedure.
      The centre of the plaster impression is given a few sharp taps to produce a crack along its crest. A cut is then made through two-thirds the depth of the impression plaster and approximately 5 mm from the posterior buccal edge. The blade of a wax knife is inserted into the cut and twisted to displace this section of the impression. The process is repeated until the impression has been removed from

the buccal aspect of the cast. The palatal area can normally be removed by placing the knife blade at the posterior junction of cast and impression and prising them apart. High rugae occasionally make this difficult, in which case the impression is removed by chipping away, piece by piece. The lingual aspect of a lower is always removed in pieces, extreme care being taken in the anterior region where a delicate ridge could be fractured.

Zinc oxide–eugenol paste

After removing the box, the cast is placed in water at 60°C for about 5 minutes. This softens the impression paste to facilitate its removal. The tray is given a sharp vertical pull which should also remove the impression material from the cast. Overheating should be avoided because it causes the impression paste to become semi-fluid in consistency and difficult to remove from the cast. In such cases the zinc oxide–eugenol paste is removed by use of a solvent such as Krex.

Hydrocolloids and elastomers

After removal of the box, the tray is given a strong vertical pull. Rotation of the tray is to be avoided because of the likelihood of damage to the underlying cast.

Master casts

Master casts are trimmed in the manner described for preliminary casts. The master cast should not be used during the construction of dental appliances but should be duplicated and the work carried out on the duplicate cast. The accuracy of the appliance may then be checked by fitting it to the master cast.

2 Cast Duplication

Various types of appliance may be constructed for fitting in the oral cavity, in the main, those used to restore or improve appearance, speech, masticatory function and lost teeth are called dentures. A denture which replaces teeth in a partially dentate mouth is referred to as a partial denture whereas the term full denture is used to describe those fitted to an edentulous mouth.

Before a denture is constructed, the cast should be analysed with a view to utilizing, to the maximum, the retentive form present in the mouth and to establish a possible path for insertion of the denture. Undercuts which may prevent insertion are eliminated. The cast is then duplicated and the denture constructed on the duplicate cast with the knowledge that the finished denture should fit the mouth.

THE PARALLELOMETER

The piece of equipment used to analyse a cast is called a parallelometer and analysing is carried out by use of an analysing rod. Analysis determines, the maximum number of parallel surfaces which may be used to enable easy insertion of a denture, position of the most bulbous areas around teeth and tissue, the depth and area of undercuts present, and finally the presence of undercuts which cannot be utilized for retention. Edentulous and partially dentate casts are analysed.

There are many types of parallelometer, some sophisticated, but most conforming to a simple design (Fig. 2.1). They consist of:
1   A solid metal base.
2   A vertical column at 90° to the base.
3   A horizontal arm, cantilevered at a right-angle to the top of the

22

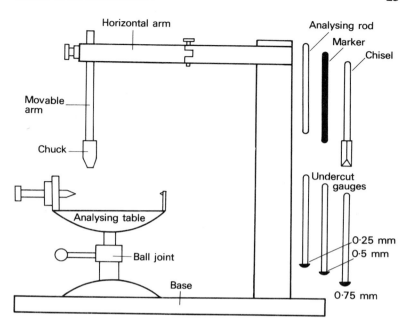

Fig. 2.1 A parallelometer.

vertical column and parallel to the base. This may be rigidly fixed to the column, free to move through 360° in a horizontal plane or on a ratchet which allows anteroposterior movement. The arm may be rigid throughout its length or be hinged at various points to allow left and right movement. Although lateral movement is helpful during the analysing procedure, the joints may eventually wear, introducing inaccuracies into the technique.

4 Suspended from the end of the horizontal arm is a movable vertical arm which is parallel to the vertical column. Its lower end contains a chuck for holding various instruments. It is generally adjustable and some are made in two halves, the lower section being spring loaded.

5 Instruments which are used in the chuck are an analysing rod, undercut gauges, chisels and a carbon marker.

6 A table (termed the analysing table) on to which the cast is secured in readiness for the analysing procedure. It is generally attached to a ball joint which allows tilting of the table. The lower half of the table may be fixed to the base of the parallelometer or have a flat base to allow freedom of movement.

CAST ANALYSIS

1   The cast is placed on the analysing table with the alveolar ridge, occlusal surface or incisal edge of the teeth in a horizontal plane, parallel to the base of the parallelometer. The analysing table should be level with the operator's eyes.

2   An analysing rod is secured in the chuck, then placed against the cast. Undercut areas will be evident by the presence of light between the rod and cast (Fig. 2.2[1]). A mental note is made of them.

3   The analysing table is initially given an anteroposterior tilt, then left and right lateral tilts and analysed in each position. The degree of tilt is altered whilst the operator looks for the maximum number of parallel surfaces which may act as guides during insertion of the denture, yet at the same time offer resistance to displacement of the denture during function. The amount of tilt given to the table is governed by the following factors.

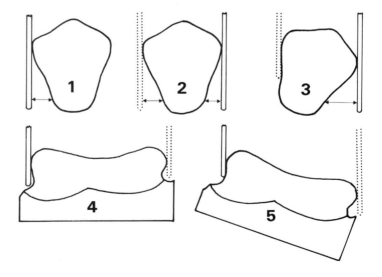

Fig. 2.2   1, undercut areas will be evident by the presence of light between the analysing rod and the cast; 2, an undercut present on both proximal surfaces of a tooth; 3, upon eliminating one undercut the other is increased; 4 and 5, elimination of an anterior tissue undercut will increase a posterior tissue undercut.

a The maximum angle to which a denture may be subjected without the teeth of the opposite jaw interfering with its insertion in the mouth.

b Elimination of an undercut by tilting of the cast should not create a problem by increasing or creating other undercuts unduly. If a tooth has an undercut on both proximal surfaces, one may be eliminated by tilting the cast but the other will be increased (Fig. 2.2[2 & 3]). Also, elimination of a tissue undercut in the anterior region may increase an undercut around the tuberosities (Fig. 2.2[4 & 5]) which would require elimination by blocking out before the denture could be inserted into the mouth. A blocked-out undercut creates a space between the denture and tissue and this results in loss of retention.

c Unless the space created between a tooth and the denture is large, food debris may stagnate in the area to cause caries or gingival inflammation. Therefore, in partial denture design the denture must either be in contact with the whole length of a tooth or be far enough away to produce an easily cleansed area.

d When a tissue undercut is increased by tilting, a space is created between the denture and tissue which reduces the retention of the denture. This is particularly relevant to full dentures which rely mainly upon natural physical forces which exist between a denture and the oral tissues for their retention (see Appendix).

It is beneficial to equalize tissue undercuts. On average the soft oral tissues is capable of being displaced by up to 0·5 mm which means only undercuts greater than this need be blocked out. In general, anterior undercuts are eliminated by altering the tilt of a cast whilst posterior ones are blocked out. This allows a denture to be inserted and seated into the mouth anterior area first.

e Tilting of the table determines the type of flexible mechanical aid (clasp) which may be incorporated in a partial denture design (see Chapter 5). As the cast is tilted, the position of the bulbous area on a tooth alters relative to the analysing rod (Fig. 2.3). If a carbon marker is exchanged for the analysing rod and lines drawn on a tooth at different tilts, it would be found that the lines would range from being near the occlusal surface to being near the gingival margin and that the angle of the line to the long axis of the tooth would also alter (Fig. 2.3). This has led to a classification of 'survey lines' (Blatterfein's classification) which is shown in Fig. 5.7 (see p. 70). The types of clasp which may be used with each line are illustrated in Chapter 5, (Figs. 5.10 and 5.11).

4 Once analysis is complete, a mental note is kept of the results of the various possible tilts and the analysing rod exchanged for an undercut guage (Fig. 2.4). There are three gauges, each with a specific use.

a 0·25 mm: used to indicate depth of undercut appropriate for cobalt chromium clasps.
b 0·5 mm: used to indicate depth of undercut appropriate for cast gold alloy clasps and maximum tissue displacement.
c 0·75 mm: used to indicate depth of undercut appropriate for wrought alloy clasps.

The teeth and tissue are reanalysed using an undercut gauge. The head of the gauge is taken to the maximum depth of the undercut

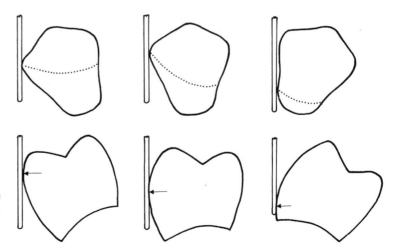

Fig. 2.3 As the cast is tilted the position of the bulbous area of a tooth alters relative to the analysing rod.

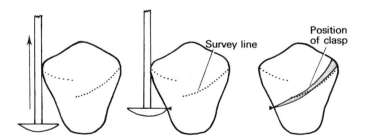

Fig. 2.4 The undercut gauge is raised until it contacts the tooth. This point indicates the position of the tip of the clasp.

and its shaft placed against the cast. The gauge is then raised until its head comes into contact with the cast which indicates the position of that particular depth of undercut (Fig. 2.4). These are noted for each of the tilts previously studied.

5 Final analysis is carried out, bearing in mind the principles of denture design.

6 Once the path of insertion has been decided upon, the analysing table is locked in position. A chisel is then placed in the chuck and three vertical grooves cut into the walls of the base of the cast, one on the left, another on the right and a final one on the posterior perpendicular wall. These indicate the angle of the cast to the horizontal plane and are used to relocate the cast, should it be removed from the parallelometer.

7 A carbon marker is next used to outline the position of maximum convexity of tooth and tissue contour.

8 Finally the protruding edge of an undercut gauge is blackened with pencil lead, and the depth of the undercut marked on the cast.

Elimination of unwanted undercuts

The cast is now ready for elimination of unwanted undercuts. Special blocking-out wax exhibiting adhesive and carving properties is normally used when the cast is to be duplicated and plaster of Paris is used when duplication is not necessary.

1 The cast is removed from the analysing table and blocking-out material placed to excess in the undercut to the level of the survey line.

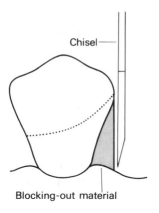

Chisel

Blocking-out material

Fig. 2.5 A chisel is used to trim the blocking-out material flush with the survey line.

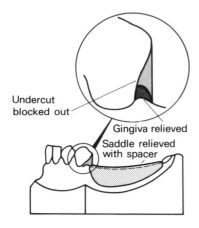

Undercut blocked out

Gingiva relieved

Saddle relieved with spacer

Fig. 2.6 A spacer is adapted to the saddle area of a partial denture when a metal structure is to have acrylic resin next to the tissue. The gingiva area is relieved and the undercut blocked.

2 The cast is returned to the analysing table and checked for correct alignment. A chisel is secured in the chuck, and used to trim the blocking-out material carefully until its blade rests on the material and survey line simultaneously (Fig. 2.5). Care should be taken to prevent damage to the cast.

PREPARATION OF CASTS

Partially dentate casts

Saddles

When a partial denture is to be made of metal with acrylic resin between the metal and tissue in the saddle area, provision must be made, during the construction of the metal for the inclusion of acrylic resin at a later stage. A 0·5 mm thick spacer of wax or tin foil is used. The saddle area of the cast is coated with a thin film of sticky wax and the spacer adapted over it. The spacer is trimmed to the design drawn on the cast. The tuberosity and retromolar pad areas are not covered with metal because it may interfere with the positioning of teeth later, therefore the spacer is terminated at the anterior border of these areas (Fig. 2.6).

Gingival margins

When a denture is so designed that it covers the gingiva, this area of the cast is relieved to prevent the denture base exerting pressure on it. This is done by filling the gingival crevice of the cast with blocking-out wax until about 0·25 mm above the gingival contour (Fig. 2.6).

Peripheral seal

To obtain retention from the natural physical forces present in the mouth (see Appendix), there must be a seal around the whole periphery of a denture. This is achieved by thickening the posterior border of a full upper denture for an edentulous mouth, and by thickening the periphery of the palatal components of an upper partial denture, so that the denture exerts light pressure on the oral tissues. The periphery of lower dentures is not thickened. The denture design is drawn on the cast, and a sharp pointed instrument used to cut a half-round shaped groove approximately 0·5 mm deep by 1·0 mm wide, from saddle area to saddle area (Fig. 2.7). When a denture terminates at the junction of the hard and soft palates, the posterior border is thickened in the manner described for full dentures (see p. 31).

A peripheral groove must not:

1   cut across the gingival tissue;
2   cut across rugae;
3   be of greater dimensions than those indicated above.

Relief of the bony areas

Bony areas, such as a torus palatinous, or torus mandibularis, should be relieved to prevent pressure from the denture. The lingual alveolar bone of the lower jaw should be relieved when a lingual bar is incorporated in the design (see Chapter 5).

Sheet casting wax is used when the cast is to be duplicated and tin foil is used when duplication is not necessary.

1   The area to be relieved is thinly coated with sticky wax.
2   The relief material, which should be about 0·2 mm thick, is cut to

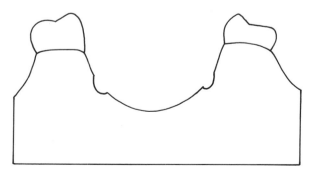

Fig. 2.7 A peripheral groove is scribed into the cast.

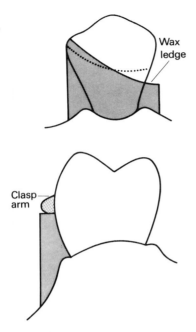

Fig. 2.8 A ledge is formed along the gingival outline of the clasp.

shape, the sticky wax softened and the relief material closely adapted to the cast. The periphery of the material is sealed with wax.

Ledges

When clasps are to be incorporated, it is advisable to transfer their proposed position to the duplicate investment cast. This is accomplished by forming a ledge along the gingival border to the intended design of the clasp. The design is drawn on the cast. Blocking-out wax is built to the gingival border of the design (Fig. 2.8) and a wax carver used to trim a perpendicular wall of wax 1 mm thick, its top edge at 90° to the wall and following the prescribed design (Fig. 2.8).

Other undercuts around standing teeth not involved in the denture design are blocked out with modelling wax to form a tapering cast from the occlusal surface to the base. This facilitates easy removal of the cast from the duplicating material.

Edentulous casts

Relief of bony areas

Bony areas should be relieved as described for partial dentures.

Edentulous ridge

When a metal denture base is to be constructed it is necessary to relieve the crest of the ridge to allow for acrylic resin to tissue contact (Fig. 2.9). The method described for partial denture saddles is used, its shape following the design features described in Chapter 5.

Rugae relief

Rugae may be relieved in the following instances:
1   When it is large and well formed.
2   When its shape is at a different angle from the path of insertion

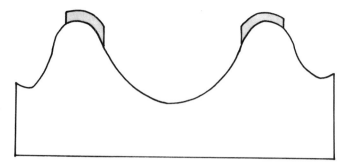

Fig. 2.9 When a metal denture is to be constructed for an edentulous patient it is necessary to relieve the crest of the alveolar ridge to allow for acrylic resin to tissue contact.

of the denture. Relief is obtained by covering with a thin film of wax. The rugae only are covered and not the areas between.

Peripheral seal

The position of the posterior border of a full upper denture is determined from oral examination by the dental surgeon. It is normally situated on the hard palate where the tissue thickness increases as it develops into the soft palate. It is often seen as a slight rise towards the posterior border of the cast (Fig. 2.10). A seal is formed by the denture exerting slight pressure on the tissue in this area and is known as the post dam.

1   The border of the denture is marked on the cast.
2   A groove about 1·5 mm deep by 1 mm wide is cut into the cast along the drawn line.
3   The anterior border of the groove is chamfered to produce a gentle slope about 3 mm wide (Fig. 2.10). This allows limited adjustment of the posterior border of the denture without the loss of the seal.

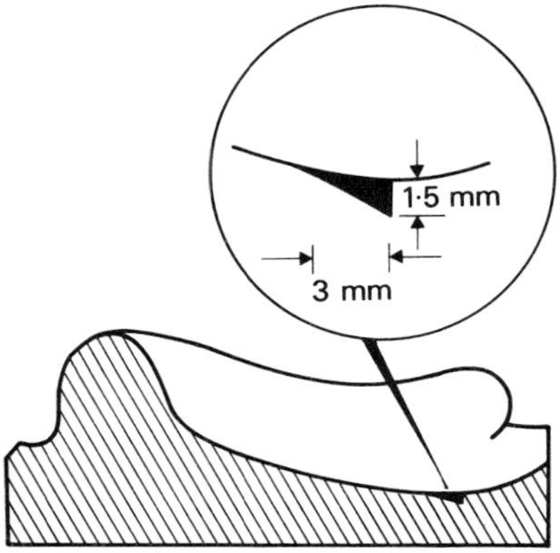

Fig. 2.10 A chamfered groove is cut into the cast, along the proposed posterior border of the denture.

DUPLICATE CASTS

Master casts should be preserved throughout all technical procedures to allow the finished appliance to be checked before insertion in the mouth. This necessitates duplication of the cast in a material appropriate for the procedure to be carried out; plaster of

Paris, dental stone, investment (see Chapter 7), or wax (see Chapter 11) may be used. An impression is taken of the cast in a hydrocolloid which has been prepared specially for duplication purposes and is known as duplicating impression material. The impression is referred to as a duplicate mould.

Before duplication, the cast is soaked in water for 15–30 minutes. This prevents a dry cast absorbing water from the duplicating material, which would affect its physical properties. It is soaked in cold water when irreversible hydrocolloid duplicating materials are to be used (a warm cast would accelerate the set of the impression material) and tepid water when reversible hydrocolloid duplicating material is to be used (a cold cast would cause the impression material to gel quickly).

Irreversible hydrocolloid mould

A duplicating flask for this material consists of a base with a lip around its edge, a D-shaped cylinder, 5 cm high, and a lid similar to the base but with three holes in its surface. The cylinder fits inside the base and lid (Fig. 2.11).

1   Excess water is dried off the surface of the presoaked master cast, which is placed in the centre of the base of the flask and sealed in position by pressing a 3 mm roll of Plasticine around it. The cylinder is positioned on the base.

2   The duplicating material is added to cold water in the proportions recommended by the manufacturer (equal parts water to powder is typical) and gently spatulated using a hand spatulator for $1\frac{1}{2}$ minutes; the mix appears slightly lumpy. It is poured into the posterior corner of the flask to allow it to slowly cover the cast without trapping air. When the flask has been filled, the lid is pressed on to the cylinder, excess material escaping through the holes.

3   After approximately 20 minutes, the base of the flask is removed to expose the cast. Removal of the Plasticine allows the fingertips to grip the sides of the cast and with a slight to and fro movement release it from the mould. Alternatively, the lid may be

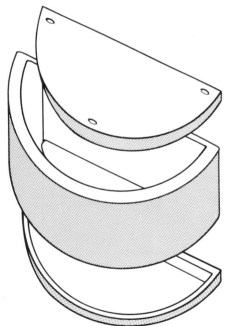

Fig. 2.11 A flask used in conjunction with an irreversible hydrocolloid duplicating material.

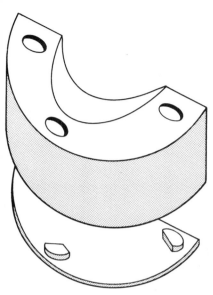

removed and the mould taken out of the flask; to and fro movement is again used to free the cast, which is lifted out of the mould. The flask and outer surface of the mould must be clean when reassembled to prevent distortion of the mould. The lid is replaced on the flask.

Reversible hydrocolloid mould

Reversible hydrocolloids require a different flask, consisting of a base and D-shaped box, the top of which has three holes, two large holes for pouring purposes and a smaller one which acts as an air vent (Fig. 2.12).

1　After drying, the presoaked cast is sealed on the base with Plasticine, the cylinder assembled on the base and the join between base and cylinder sealed with Plasticine, or a large elastic band. This prevents the fluid reversible hydrocolloid from leaking out of the flask.

2　When a small quantity of hydrocolloid is required it is heated in a double pan; when a large quantity is required it is heated in a thermostatically controlled electric bath with dispensing facilities. A temperature of 90°C is required to melt the hydrocolloid but it does not commence to gel until 45°C. This factor is called hysteresis.

3　The fluid hydrocolloid is cooled and its temperature is checked with a thermometer. When the temperature falls to 50–55°C the fluid hydrocolloid is poured into the flask through one of the large holes until excess material appears at the other holes. It is allowed to cool on the bench for at least 30 minutes, then placed in approximately 10 mm of cold water to quicken the cooling process; complete immersion may cause distortion of the mould. One hour after pouring, the base of the flask and the Plasticine around the master cast are removed, as is excess hydrocolloid around the lip of the flask. Slight pressure on the hydrocolloid through the holes in the flask releases the mould. Excess material around the area of the pouring holes is cut away and a rocking movement used to release the cast which is lifted out of the mould. The mould is checked for accuracy of detail and possible damage, then returned to the flask.

Fig. 2.12　A flask used in conjunction with a reversible hydrocolloid duplicating material.

Pouring the cast

A solution of potassium sulphate, an accelerator of the setting of calcium sulphate, is poured into the mould to saturate the surface of the hydrocolloid. This counteracts the retarding effect that the exudate of the hydrocolloid has upon the setting of calcium sulphate. Prolonged soaking results in distortion, therefore, the solution is left in the mould for 1 minute only, then poured off. The use of potassium sulphate is recommended only when pouring plaster of Paris and dental stone. The cast is poured in the manner already described in Chapter 1.

When the cast reaches its initial set (see Appendix), the mould is placed in a humidor (see Appendix) or a damp cloth placed over the exposed surface, to prevent evaporation of water from the mould. The cast is allowed to set for 1 hour.

Removal from the mould

1   Mould and cast are removed from the flask as an integral unit.
2   A series of cuts, two-thirds the depth of the hydrocolloid, is made around the mould about 20 mm apart, care being taken not to score the cast. Each section is peeled off the cast, followed by the centre section which is normally removed in one piece.
3   Irreversible duplicating materials are discarded whilst reversible ones are washed and sealed in an airtight container to prevent loss of water. The flask is cleaned.
4   The base of the cast only is trimmed. Water should not be used when trimming investment duplicate casts but the machine should be flushed with water immediately after use to prevent blockage.

Investment duplicate cast

Investment materials are explained briefly in Chapter 6. The surface of an investment cast is rather soft and frail when compared with dental stone, especially those bonded by calcium sulphate. The surface can be damaged easily when carrying out a technical procedure. It is impregnated with a resin to strengthen it.

1   The trimmed investment cast is placed in an oven, the temperature of which is raised to 130°C over 1 hour.

2   Meanwhile the resin is heated until completely fluid.

3   The cast is placed on a cradle immersed in the fluid for about 15 seconds, then taken out and drained for 15 seconds. This is repeated until the total immersion time is 1 minute. The excess is poured off, and the cast bench cooled. It is then ready for use.

3 Occlusal Rims and Bases

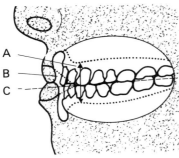

Fig. 3.1 A, vertical dimension; B, relationship between labial surface of anterior teeth and the lips; C, occlusal plane.

If a patient is to obtain maximum benefit from an appliance, it must harmonize with the oral environment. This demands recording specific information from the oral cavity for use in the laboratory. A cast records details of the natural dentition and alveolar ridges but the following information is also required before dentures can be constructed.

1 Centric relation; the static relationship between maxilla and mandible when the condyles are in their most retruded position in the glenoid fossae at the correct vertical dimension.

2 Vertical dimension; the distance between the alveolar process of the maxilla and mandible when in centric relation (Fig. 3.1).

3 The occlusal plane; the position and angle of a plane to which the occlusal surfaces of teeth relate (Fig. 3.1).

4 Labial contour; the relationship between the labial surface of the anterior teeth and lips (Fig. 3.1).

5 The centre line; this indicates the centre of the patient's face (Fig. 3.2).

6 Normal lip line; this indicates the rest position of the upper lip and may be 2–3 mm higher than the occlusal plane.

7 High lip line; the position of the upper lip when the patient smiles (Fig. 3.2).

8 Corner or canine lines; the position of the corner of the mouth (Fig. 3.2). This indicates the approximate centre of the incisal edge of the upper canines.

9 The muscular neutral zone (the zone of equilibrium); where the forces from the muscles of the face and tongue are equal and opposite. The position of teeth in the natural dentition is determined by this muscular activity. An appliance situated in the mouth is also subject to the same muscular activity which can displace it unless the replacing teeth are placed in the neutral zone. Unfortu-

36

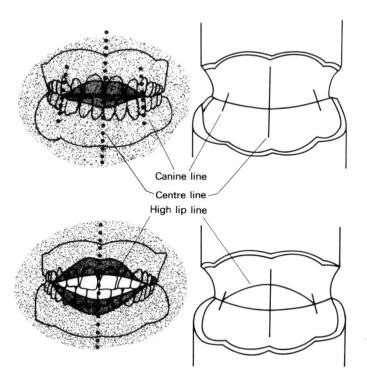

Canine line
Centre line
High lip line

Fig. 3.2 Oral information recorded on occlusal rims and bases.

nately, the edentulous ridge does undergo resorption upon loss of teeth, and therefore does not indicate the position of the neutral zone.

Some of this information is recorded on a dentate cast, but when teeth are missing their positions are taken by blocks and the information recorded on these. The blocks are attached to a base constructed to accurately fit the mouth. Jointly, they are termed record or registration blocks, but occlusal rim and base is more descriptive and will be used throughout this book.

The occlusal rim and base, with its associated information, is a functional prescription. It is also accompanied by a written prescription, both of which are essential when an appliance is to be constructed in the absence of the patient. Much chairside time can be eliminated if the rim is constructed to the size and shape of the natural dentition. Study casts, poured before extraction of the teeth, are helpful for this purpose. When such casts are not available, the operator must rely upon experience and knowledge of oral anatomy combined with information obtainable from the edentulous cast.

ANATOMICAL INFORMATION

Maxilla

1   The labial surface of anterior teeth support the lips and this position should be maintained if there is to be no major change in the patient's facial profile. On average, the labial surface of the centrals is between 10 and 12 mm labial of a slight oval rise in the palatal tissue called the incisive papilla (Fig. 3.3). Upon extraction of teeth major resorption takes place on the labial surface of the alveolar process but the incisive papilla remains. This may be used to indicate the position of the labial surface of the centrals (Fig. 3.4).

2   The centre of the last molar is approximately opposite the centre of the tuberosity and its buccal surface between 3 and 5 mm buccal of the centre of the tuberosity (Fig. 3.5). Upon extraction of teeth the major resorption takes place on the buccal wall of the alveolar

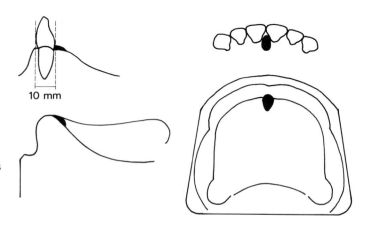

10 mm

Fig. 3.3   The position of the incisive papilla on an edentulous cast and its relationship to the labial surface of the natural dentition.

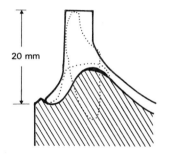

Fig. 3.4 The major resorption takes place on the labial surface of the alveolar process leaving the incisive papilla in the region of the crest of the ridge. The distance from the functional sulcus to the incisal edge of the centrals is around 20 mm.

ridge which sometimes results in a buccally protrusive tuberosity (Fig. 3.5). The centre of the tuberosity gives some indication of the position of the posterior teeth.

3 The length of a tooth gives no indication of the amount of resorption likely to take place upon its extraction. However, on average, the distance from the functional sulcus to the incisal edge of the centrals is 20 mm (Fig. 3.4). The distance from the sulcus to the occlusal surface of the first molar is about 18 mm. These dimensions indicate the approximate height of the occlusal plane.

Mandible

1 There is no specific area from which the position of the labial surface of lower anterior teeth may be estimated, but most resorption takes place on the labial surface of the alveolar ridge.

2 The centre of the last molar is buccal of the retromolar pad by about 3 mm. Resorption of the alveolar bone in the posterior segments may be considered as being in a vertical direction (although not true in all cases), from which it may be surmised that on average, the centre of the ridge approximates with the centre of the posterior teeth.

3 The vertical height of teeth from the functional sulcus to the incisal edge of the centrals is about the same as the upper dimensions. The occlusal surface of posterior teeth corresponds, on average, with the centre of the retromolar pad.

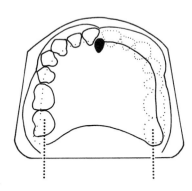

Fig. 3.5 The centre of the last molar is approximately opposite the centre of the tuberosity. The major resorption takes place on the buccal wall of the alveolar process.

BASES

Ideally, a material used to form a base should be easy to handle, capable of reproducing detail from the cast and should not distort at mouth temperature. It should also be capable of being modified at the chairside by additions or trimming as well as being compatible with materials used to form the rim. Materials used are modelling wax, shellac, acrylic resin and impression compound.

Bases for edentulous mouths

Wax base

Modelling wax tends to distort if left in the mouth or if submitted to a heavy occlusal force, and so wire is incorporated to minimize the distortion. The following procedures are best carried out on a duplicate cast, the master cast being preserved for further duplication in case of accident and for checking purposes.

1   The posterior palatal border of the upper base finishes at the junction of the hard and soft palates. It is marked on the cast.

2   A piece of modelling wax, sufficient to cover the cast is cut and softened over a Bunsen burner flame as described under spacers (see Chapter 2). It is adapted carefully to the palatal or lingual surface of the cast. As the wax hardens it is resoftened and adaption is continued; the palatal or lingual aspect being held firmly in position whilst being closely adapted to the buccal and labial aspect. The sulcus must be accurately reproduced and so the curved end of a slightly warmed wax knife, is used to press wax into the sulcus area.

3   The wax is trimmed to the outer edge of the sulcus and to the palatal finishing line by use of a warm wax knife.

4   A 7 cm length of 1 mm round nickel silver wire is cut and bent in the fingers to approximate the lingual or palatal contour of the alveolar ridge. Its length is adjusted to terminate at the mesial edge of the retromolar pad or tuberosity. It is positioned on the wax with its top edge about 2 mm below the crest of the ridge and sealed in position with molten modelling wax (Fig. 3.6). The handling of the wax is important. A little wax is placed on the blade of a wax knife and the handle end of the blade heated to melt the wax and confine it at the tip of the blade. The knife is then used in the fashion of a pen, the edge of the wax just touching the wire and base, and the knife moved along the join. The process is repeated until the wire is covered with an even layer of wax.

5   Wax is next made to flow into the concavity in the sulcus area and light finger-pressure applied to the solidifying wax to minimize distortion. About 0·5 mm of wax is trimmed from around all muscle

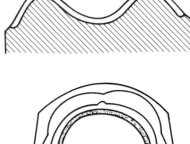
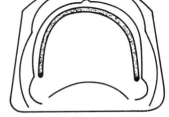

Fig. 3.6   Position of a wire strengthener.

attachments. The base is removed from the cast, its fitting surface checked for accuracy of detail and then returned to the cast.

Shellac base

This material is similar to the one used for special tray construction but is thinner, generally pink in colour and contains no filler. Shellac is more stable than wax at mouth temperature but is more difficult to adjust at the chairside. Consequently, its use is often confined to an upper palate with the buccal and labial sulcus formed in wax. A wax base with a wire insert is generally used on the lower.

1 The shellac should finish just below the crest of the ridge and at the junction of hard and soft palates (Fig. 3.7). This position is drawn on the cast which is then dusted lightly with French chalk to prevent shellac sticking to it.

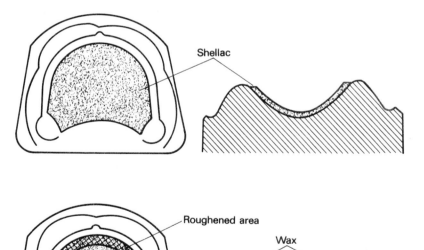

Fig. 3.7 The shellac is finished just below the crest of the ridge and a 5 mm band roughened. Wax is adapted to the sulcus and to the shellac.

2   The shellac is softened in the manner described for special trays and adapted to the palate, care being taken to prevent thinning.

3   Its periphery is resoftened and trimmed to a general shape by the use of scissors. Final shaping is accomplished by use of a file, the edge of the shellac being chamfered to blend into the ridge. It may need further heating and adaption before the edges are smoothed with sandpaper. Retentive form, for attachment of the rim is made by roughening the shellac with a hot wax knife in the form of a 5 mm wide band and coating it lightly with sticky wax (Fig. 3.7).

4   A strip of modelling wax, the length of the sulcus area, is softened and adapted to the sulcus, outer surface of the alveolar ridge and on to the roughened area of the shellac (Fig. 3.7). It is sealed to the shellac by use of a hot wax knife which is also used to penetrate the wax along the periphery of the shellac to seal it and to reproduce detail from the ridge. Slight finger-pressure is exerted as the wax solidifies.

5   Muscle attachments are relieved and the fitting surface of the base checked for accuracy of detail.

Impression compound base

Impression compound may be used as an alternative to shellac but it is normal to confine its use to cases where the rim is to be of the same material. It is reasonably stable at mouth temperature and can be adjusted at the chairside by use of a warm wax knife.

The impression compound is softened in a water bath at a temperature of 60°C and flattened into an arch form about 1·5 mm thick and large enough to cover the whole cast. It is resoftened, and adapted to the cast as described for wax bases. The edge may be resoftened in water or over a Bunsen burner flame to allow for trimming. A file is used for final trimming. Impression compound is easily thinned and distorted during construction of the base but is reasonably stable once shaped.

Acrylic resin base

The fit and stability of heat-polymerizing and autopolymerizing acrylic resins are superior to other forms of base. Heat-polymerizing acrylic resin firstly requires the formation of a wax pattern of the base. This is used to form a mould into which the acrylic resin is compressed and then hardened (see Chapter 10). Autopolymerizing resins do not require the formation of a mould hence the technique is quicker. It is essential that autopolymerizing acrylic resin is formed on a duplicate cast with unnecessary undercut areas eliminated, otherwise difficulty may be experienced with removal of the base from the cast. The construction of an auto-polymerizing acrylic resin base will be described.

1   The duplicate cast is coated with a separating medium, such as sodium alginate.

2   About 4 cm^3 of monomer is placed in a mixing vessel and the polymer sprinkled into it until a doughy consistency is obtained. This is flattened between two pieces of Cellophane or polythene sheet to produce an arch form sufficiently large to cover the cast.

3   The Cellophane is removed and the acrylic resin adapted to the cast, care being taken to prevent thinning.

4   The periphery may be trimmed to the general shape with scissors whilst the acrylic resin is soft or left until polymerization is complete (the resin hardens), when trimming is accomplished by use of a rotating carborundum wheel on a dental lathe, followed by a rotary trimmer held in a handpiece.

5   A more accurately-fitting base may be obtained by coating the fitting surface of the base with a further layer of autopolymerizing acrylic resin.

   The cast is cleaned of sodium alginate by use of a hard brush, and then recoated with the same material. A fluid mix of acrylic resin is poured over the fitting surface of the base, the cast seated on it and held firmly in position by use of an elastic band. When polymerization is complete, the base is removed from the cast, the periphery and upper surface smoothed with sandpaper, then polished (see Chapter 10).

OCCLUSAL RIMS

Occlusal rims may be constructed in wax, impression compound,

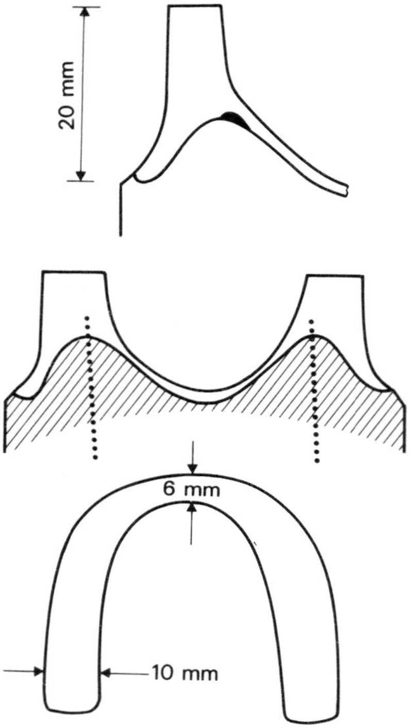

Fig. 3.8 Dimensions of a maxillary occlusal rim. The centre of its posterior region should be buccal of the centre of the alveolar ridge.

impression compound with a plaster–pumice occlusal insert or entirely of plaster of Paris and pumice. All types of rim are constructed in accordance with basic principles but these may be modified occasionally for specific clinical procedures.

Principles of occlusal rim design

Maxillary occlusal rim

1 The height of the occlusal rim from the sulcus to the occlusal surface should be approximately 20 mm in the labial region, 18 mm in the posterior region and approximately 15 mm anterior of the tuberosity (Fig. 3.8). This results in the height of the rim varying from patient to patient depending upon the resorption that has taken place.

2 The anterior width of the rim should be 6–8 mm (Fig. 3.8). Although the incisal edge of anterior teeth seldom exceeds 3 mm in width, the relationship between the upper and lower anterior teeth can vary greatly. This necessitates the rim width being increased to allow upper and lower rims to contact and offer stability during the laboratory procedure.

3 The posterior width should be 8–10 mm to ensure contact with the lower rim (Fig. 3.8).

4 On average, the labial surface of the rim should be 10 mm anterior of the incisive papilla (see p. 38, Fig. 3.3).

5 The centre of the posterior region of the occlusal rim should be 2–3 mm buccal of the centre of the alveolar ridge.

6 The posterior border of the occlusal surface should terminate on the anterior aspect of the tuberosity and the rim tapered to the base at the distal aspects of the tuberosity. This prevents interference with the ascending ramus of the mandible.

7 The walls of the occlusal rim should make a 90° angle with the occlusal surface until level with the crest of the alveolar ridge, then gradually taper to the sulcus or palate (Fig. 3.8). This shape allows maximum space for the tongue, and the curved buccal surface allows the oral musculature to stabilize the base.

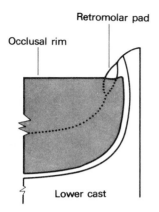

Occlusal rim

Retromolar pad

Lower cast

Fig. 3.9 The mandibular occlusal rim terminates at the centre of the retromolar pad.

Mandibular occlusal rim

1   The anterior height of the mandibular occlusal rim, from the sulcus to the occlusal surface, should be approximately 18 mm.

2   It is difficult to determine a definite dimension for the posterior region; instead, the retromolar pad is taken as the reference point, the occlusal rim being finished at the centre of the pad (Fig. 3.9).

3   The anterior width should be approximately 4–6 mm and the posterior width 6–8 mm.

4   The anterior and posterior segments of the rim are formed directly over the lower alveolar ridge.

5   The occlusal rim should terminate at the centre of the retromolar pad. Its walls should make a 90° angle with the occlusal surface until level with the crest of the alveolar ridge, then taper to the buccal and lingual sulci. The tongue and other oral musculature stabilizes the base.

   The dimensions indicated may be checked by the use of a measuring device (see Appendix).

Wax occlusal rims

Wax is used extensively in the construction of occlusal rims, mainly because it is easy to handle in the laboratory and to modify at the chairside. The wax rim may be formed in one of three ways:

1   By using a wax occlusal rim purchased from a manufacturer.

2   By pouring wax into a mould of an occlusal rim.

3   By moulding a sheet of modelling wax.

   Each rim is attached to the base in a similar manner, therefore, the last method only will be described.

1   A full sheet of modelling wax is sufficient for most cases. It is softened over a Bunsen burner flame until soft and pliable throughout, when it is bent in half and pressed closely together. Every effort is taken to prevent air inclusion between the layers.

2   It is resoftened, tightly rolled into a rod and its cross-section formed into a 12 mm square by pressing the wax between finger and thumb of both hands simultaneously. This also increases its length.

3   It is again softened and now adapted to the alveolar ridge area of the base, from tuberosity or retromolar pad on one side of the cast to the same region of the opposite side of the cast.

4   The occlusal surface is flattened against a plate (a 10 cm ceramic tile is ideal) until the required vertical height is obtained. This produces a widening of the occlusal surface and so the excess wax is pressed on to the base and sealed to it by use of a hot wax knife.

5   Discrepancies in the contour of the rim are corrected by additions of wax. These are melted on a wax knife and dripped on to the walls of the rim and base.

6   Once smooth, the dimensions of the rim are corrected by cutting and scraping, followed by the walls being smoothed by the curved end of a hot wax knife. An outward curved shape from the occlusal surface to the sulcus should be produced which allows the oral musculature to sit on the base to help retain it.

7   The occlusal rim and base is removed from the cast and the outer edge of the periphery of the base smoothed without damaging its contour. Finally, the occlusal rim and base is returned to the cast, the wax smoothed by use of a fine flame and polished by rubbing with cotton wool whilst being held under cold running water. It is removed from the cast and placed in cold water.

8   The cast is cleaned of residual wax by pouring boiling water over it. Its walls are then sandpapered smooth and dusted lightly with French chalk. The occlusal rim and base is returned to the cast, ready for presentation to the surgery.

Impression compound occlusal rim

Although more stable than wax, an impression compound occlusal rim is difficult to modify at the chairside. For this reason it is used in conjunction with a wax occlusal wafer which records the occlusal relationship, other relevant information being recorded by a wax occlusal rim and base.

The base may be constructed in impression compound or acrylic resin.

1   Sufficient impression compound is softened in water at a temperature of 60°C. It is shaped and adapted to the base in the manner described for wax.

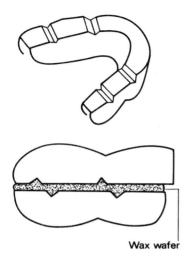

Fig. 3.10 Impression compound occlusal rim, showing localizing notches and a wax wafer.

2 The compound is sealed to the base by use of a hot wax knife, and its occlusal surface levelled. Excess material is removed with the aid of a hot wax knife and the occlusal surface reduced until 2 mm shorter than wax rims to allow space for a wax wafer. It is smoothed by use of sandpaper.

3 Four grooves are cut into the occlusal surface of each rim about 3 mm wide by 2 mm deep. One groove is cut in the last molar region, another in the first premolar region on each side of the arch (Fig. 3.10). A file is used for this purpose.

4 The occlusal rim and base is given a high gloss by flaming, followed by rubbing with a pledget of cotton wool whilst held under cold running water.

Various jaw relationships may be recorded by the use of wax wafers (see p. 49) placed between the rims. Protrusions are formed on the wafer corresponding to the notches in the occlusal rim.

Impression compound with plaster–pumice occlusal insert

The occlusal rims so far described, record a flat occlusal plane, but in nature it is spheroidal in shape consisting of an anteroposterior and lateral curvature (see Chapter 9). There are instances when it may be useful to know this curvature (see Chapter 9). It may be produced by inserting an easily abraded material into the occlusal surface of a rim and requesting the patient to perform normal jaw gliding movements with the upper and lower occlusal rims in contact. Such occlusal rims are called abrasive rims the occlusal surface being made in a mixture of plaster of Paris and pumice.

1 Although impression compound is generally used to form the rim, autopolymerizing acrylic resin is firmer and does not deform during the lengthy process. The occlusal rim is constructed in the normal manner but with a vertical dimension 2 mm shorter than normal.

2 Retentive form, is cut into the occlusal surface of the rim for securing the plaster–pumice mix. A box 3 mm deep with tapering walls in a dovetail shape is cut by use of a flat-edged sculptor (Fig. 3.11). The walls of the box should be 1·0–1·5 mm thick.

3 Equal parts of plaster of Paris and pumice are added to water

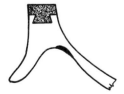

Fig. 3.11 An impression compound occlusal rim with a plaster–pumice occlusal insert.

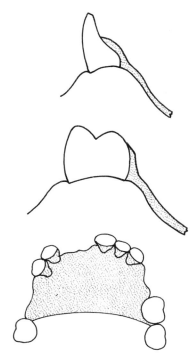

and spatulated to a creamy consistency. This is placed in the box and sufficient added to produce a 3 mm thick layer over the whole occlusal surface. The mix is allowed to set.

4 The surface is flattened and reduced to 2 mm thickness by rubbing on sandpaper. The sides of the rim are also smoothed.

It is necessary to know the patient's vertical dimension before constructing such an occlusal rim because it cannot be modified at the chairside without loss of the plaster–pumice surface. This entails recording the normal information by use of a wax occlusal rim and base at an earlier visit of the patient.

Bases for the partially dentate mouth

Shellac or autopolymerizing acrylic resin may be used for the base but although acrylic resin produces the stronger base, shellac seems to be universally used. As will be seen in Chapter 5 some bases are constructed in metal and this may also be used as the base for an occlusal rim.

1 The duplicate cast is dusted with French chalk and a piece of shellac softened and adapted to it. It is not adapted to the occlusal surface of standing teeth.

2 The shellac is resoftened and trimmed to a general shape using scissors.

3 After further softening and adaption it is removed from the cast and accurately trimmed by use of a file. It should finish above the survey line (see Chapter 2) of standing teeth in the posterior region and be contoured to sit on the cingulum of anterior teeth (Fig. 3.12). (This shape may be modified according to the designs illustrated under partial dentures (see Chapter 5) but greater stability is obtained at this stage by using the method described.)

4 A wire insert should be incorporated in a lower base. A piece of 1 mm nickel silver wire is bent to conform to the shape of the alveolar ridge, warmed and embedded into the surface of the shellac. (It must not penetrate the shellac.) It is sealed to the base with sticky wax then covered with modelling wax.

5 The occlusal rim is formed according to the principles described,

Fig. 3.12 Adapting shellac to a partially dentate cast. Shellac is adapted to the cingulum of anterior teeth and above the survey line on posterior teeth.

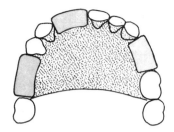

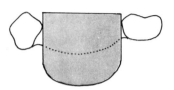

Fig. 3.13 An occlusal rim should not protrude above standing teeth and be no wider than the abutment teeth.

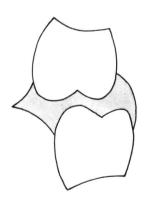

Fig. 3.14 A wax wafer registration, illustrating the buccal ridge formed to strengthen the registration.

the standing teeth being used as a guide for its position and height (Fig. 3.13). It should not protrude above the occlusal surface of standing teeth or be wider than them. The base and rim are smoothed and polished in the manner described.

WAFER REGISTRATIONS

Jaw relationships of dentate and some partially dentate mouths are recorded by taking an impression of the occlusal surfaces of the teeth. The impression is thin in section and is termed a wafer registration. They are also used in conjunction with compound rims. Wax, irreversible hydrocolloid, plaster of Paris and zinc oxide–eugenol paste may be used. Details for taking these registrations are given in textbooks on clinical dentistry.

Wax wafer registration

Modelling wax or special wax containing aluminium powder may be used. A strip, the length of the occlusal table and about 5 cm wide is softened and a piece of dental napkin or Cellophane about 1·5 cm wide laid along one side. The wax is wrapped around the Cellophane to form a double thickness on one side and single thickness on the other. This is resoftened then placed in the mouth and the registration taken. Excess wax buccally and labially is formed into a ridge to strengthen the registration and prevent distortion (Fig. 3.14). Wax wafer registrations should be kept cool until required for use.

Alternative wafer registrations

Plaster of Paris, zinc oxide–eugenol paste and irreversible hydrocolloids are all used in the same manner. A wire frame, the size of the occlusal table, is made from 1·5–2·0 mm nickel silver or stainless steel wire. A piece of dental gauze is stretched over the wire and attached to it by use of sticky wax. This secures the material to the wire frame, but does not interfere with the occlusion during the registration procedure. The material is placed on both sides of the gauze to a thickness of 2 mm and the jaw relationship recorded. Irreversible hydrocolloid wafer impressions should be placed in a suitable humidor until required for use.

4 Articulators

The information obtained from casts and occlusal rims and bases may be termed static information, but the mouth is a dynamic system. Therefore, some means should be available in the laboratory for converting static information into a dynamic form and this is done by mounting the casts on an instrument called an articulator. Basically, it consists of two arms, to which casts of the maxilla and mandible are attached, interlocked at a movable joint representing the temporomandibular joint (TMJ). The ideal articulator should

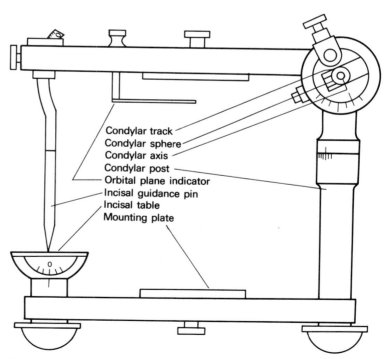

Condylar track
Condylar sphere
Condylar axis
Condylar post
Orbital plane indicator
Incisal guidance pin
Incisal table
Mounting plate

Fig. 4.1 Fully adjustable anatomical articulator (based on the Dentatus articulator).

51

possess means of adjustment to an individual patient's requirements. Such an articulator is the fully adjustable anatomical articulator (Fig. 4.1), but special information, not recorded by occlusal rims and bases is required to enable the articulator to be adjusted (see p. 54).

A less sophisticated form of this articulator is the fixed condylar path or average value anatomical articulator. This incorporates the basic movements of the TMJ but they have been calculated to be that of the average patient. Generally speaking, they are capable of minor adjustment only (Fig. 4.2).

The simplest articulator is the plane line or simple hinge (Fig. 4.3), which allows opening and closing movements only. Although perhaps the most widely used in the commercial world, it essentially establishes static oral information and takes no account of the dynamic environment of the oral cavity. Its usefulness can be improved by the use of plaster–pumice blocks (see p. 157).

Unlike the oral mechanism the upper arm of the articulator moves and not the lower. The articulator is so designed for ease of handling. Therefore it will be seen that mandibular movements

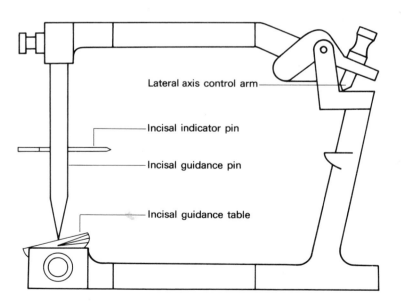

Lateral axis control arm

Incisal indicator pin

Incisal guidance pin

Incisal guidance table

Fig. 4.2 Fixed condylar path articulator (based on the New Simplex articulator).

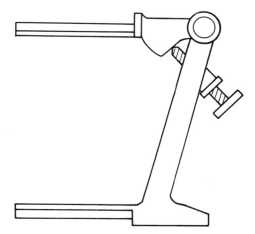

Fig. 4.3 Plane line or simple hinge articulator.

are translated into the movements on the articulator shown in Table 4.1.

Table 4.1 Comparison of natural and articulated movements.

Mandibular movement	*Articulator movement*
Protrusive	The upper arm moves in a posterior direction
Right lateral	The upper arm moves to the left
Left lateral	The upper arm moves to the right

The articulator is held with the incisor region facing the operator, in the manner of looking at a patient's face. A movement to the patient's right will be seen by the operator as a movement to the left. A patient's lateral movements will therefore be seen by the operator as shown in Table 4.2

Table 4.2 Apparent movements on articulator.

Mandibular movement	*Articulator movement*	*Seen by operator*
Right lateral	Movement to the left	Movement to the right
Left lateral	Movement to the right	Movement to the left

FULLY ADJUSTABLE ANATOMICAL ARTICULATOR

Besides the information recorded by occlusal rims and bases or wafer registrations, further information in the form of the relationship between maxilla and the condyles is required before casts can be mounted on a fully adjustable anatomical articulator. This relationship is recorded by use of a face bow (Fig. 4.4), which is a U-shaped frame with a movable rod at the end of each of its arms. These are positioned over the patient's condyles whilst a smaller U-shaped frame, called a bite fork and attached to the bow, is used to record the occlusal surface of the upper standing teeth or occlusal rim. A further attachment, the orbital pin, is used to indicate the position of the orbital plane which relates the angle of the occlusal plane to an imaginary horizontal plane from the condyles to the orbital arch, the Frankfort plane. The face bow is used to transfer the maxillary-condylar relationship to the articulator.

Separate upper and lower occlusal rims and bases (often made from impression compound with a wax wafer) are used to record centric relation which is required for mounting the lower cast on to the articulator. Wafer registrations are used when dentate casts are to be mounted.

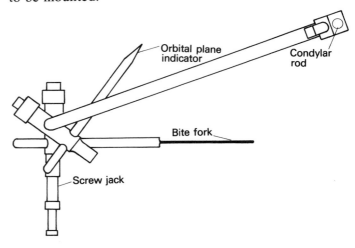

Fig. 4.4 A face bow.

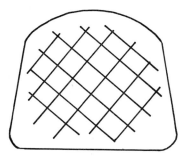

Fig. 4.5 The base of each cast is deeply scored to produce a key into which the mounting plaster will interlock.

1   The base of each cast is deeply scored by use of a sharp knife to produce a key into which the mounting plaster will interlock (Fig. 4.5). They are soaked in a bowl of cold water for about 15 minutes. Failure to carry out this procedure will result in a dry cast absorbing water from the mounting plaster which will impair the bond between new and old plaster.

2   The movable sections of the articulator are adjusted (Fig. 4.6):

    a   Condylar posts are set to 15°.
    b   Condylar tracks are set to 40°.
    c   Condylar axis and its sphere is set to its basic central position.
    d   Incisal guidance pin is set to zero.
    e   Incisal guidance table is set to zero degrees and horizontal when viewed from all sides.
    f   The orbital plane indicator is attached to the upper arm of the articulator.
    g   All locking screws are secured.
    h   Mounting discs are lightly lubricated and secured to the articulator.

3   The upper cast is secured with wax to either the occlusal wafer or occlusal rim and base, attached to the bite fork.

4   The calibrated movable condylar rods on the face bow are positioned on the condylar axis of the articulator. The calibrations will have been equalized by the surgeon during the clinical procedures.

5   A jack screw, attached to the bite fork securing device, is adjusted to raise the anterior region of the face bow to raise the orbital pin until it contacts the orbital plane indicator.

6   The upper arm is rotated to the rear of the articulator. Plaster of Paris is mixed with water to a creamy consistency, a large increment placed on the base of the upper cast and the upper arm of the articulator rotated forwards and pressed into the plaster (Fig. 4.6). It is important that the incisal guidance pin contacts the incisal table. Great care should be exercised to prevent displacement of the bite fork or face bow. A supporting block of plaster may be helpful. More plaster is added to the top of the mounting disc.

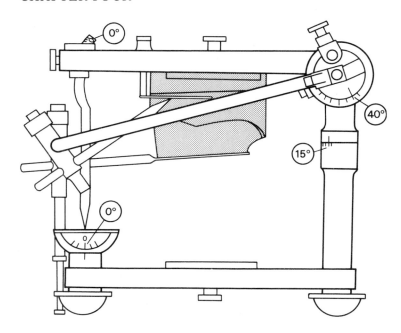

Fig. 4.6 Mounting the upper cast on a fully adjustable articulator with the aid of a face bow.

7   Once the mounting plaster has set, the face bow and its attachments are removed from the articulator and the mounting plaster trimmed.

8   An occlusal rim and base or occlusal wafer, recording centric relation is secured to the upper cast, and the lower cast or occlusal rim secured to it.

9   The articulator is inverted with the upper arm sitting on the plaster bench, whilst the lower cast is secured to the mounting disc with plaster of Paris in the manner described for the upper. The incisal guidance pin must contact the incisal table.

10 After trimming, the mounting plaster is smoothed with sandpaper and the articulator cleaned of plaster debris.

Adjustment of the articulator

The following information is required when adjusting the articulator to the individual patient's condylar movements.

1   Relation of the mandible to the maxilla in protrusive excursion. Together with the centric relation record, this allows the condylar angles and forward condylar movement to be transferred to the articulator.

2   Relation of the mandible to the maxilla in left and right lateral excursions. These records provide a more individual estimate of each condylar angle and also give an indication of the degree of the Bennett shift (see p. 149).

These are recorded by the use of wafer registrations, but both are not necessarily required; in fact some patients are unable to make lateral excursions even with their teeth apart.

Using a protrusive registration

The protrusive registration wafer is used to adjust the condylar angle or horizontal condylar inclination.

1   The locking nuts to the condylar spheres and condylar tracks are released and the incisal guidance pin is raised in its housing and locked off the incisal table.

2   The protrusive registration wafer is placed on the lower cast or occlusal rim and the upper cast or occlusal rim carefully seated into it by moving the upper arm of the articulator bodily in a posterior direction.

3   Gentle pressure is exerted to the centre of the upper arm of the articulator whilst first one and then the other condylar track is rotated to and fro until the cast or occlusal rim seats evenly in the registration. The locking nut of each track is tightened in turn, followed by the locking nuts of the condylar spheres.

4   The new calibrations recorded on the condylar tracks are noted on the laboratory prescription form, for reference should the settings be altered.

Using lateral registrations

These are used to adjust the condylar pillars which govern the lateral condylar angle or the inward angle of movement of the condyles when the jaw moves to the left or right.

1 The lock nut to the condylar pillar opposite to the direction of movement is loosened and the pillar turned to its highest calibration. Consequently, the right pillar is loosened when the articulator is to move to the left.

2 The appropriate wafer registration is positioned on the lower cast and the upper seated into the registration. The pillar is rotated to a smaller calibration whilst light pressure is exerted to the upper arm of the articulator, until the upper cast seats evenly into the registration. The pillar is then secured in its new position by tightening the lock nut and the registration removed.

3 The process is repeated with the second lateral registration and the opposite pillar adjusted. A note is made of the new calibrations registered by the condylar pillars.

4 Finally, the horizontal condylar inclination is checked to ensure that no alteration has been introduced by the lateral adjustments.

All the wafer registrations are stored for future reference. The incisal guidance pin is lowered to the incisal table and locked in position. Adjustments may be made to the incisal table, but this will be dealt with in Chapter 9.

AVERAGE VALUE ARTICULATOR

There are various types of average value articulator but the principle behind their use is similar to the adjustable types. Some have facilities for the use of a face bow, but generally, the relationship of maxilla to the condyles is established by aligning the occlusal surface of the upper occlusal rim with the incisal pin and with notches or a bar at the rear of the articulator.

1 The base of the casts are scored, the occlusal rims checked to ensure they are sealed together and the casts seated in the bases. These are formed into an integral unit by two wax strips placed either side of the casts. A 2 cm wide strip of modelling wax, about 2 cm longer than the distance between the bases of the casts is softened and adapted to the premolar region. Approximately 1 cm of wax is bent on to the base of each cast and sealed to it (Fig. 4.7).

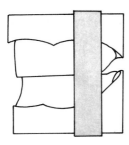

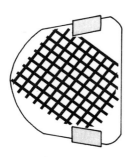

Fig. 4.7 The casts are bound together by use of two strips of wax.

The whole unit is then placed in cold water for 15 minutes to allow the casts to absorb water.

2 The mounting areas of both arms of the articulator are lightly lubricated.

3 The following movable parts of the articulator are adjusted:

    a Lateral axis control arms, when present, are set in their outermost position (Fig. 4.8).

    b The incisal guidence pin is set flush with the top of the pin housing on the upper arm of the articulator (Fig. 4.8).

    c The incisal indicator pin is located in the incisal guidance pin (Fig. 4.8). The head of the incisal indicator pin must be firmly against the incisal guidance pin.

    d The incisal guidance table is set to zero degrees. (horizontal) (Fig. 4.8).

4 Three small pillars of Plasticine are placed in a triangular formation on the lower arm of the articulator and the base of the lower

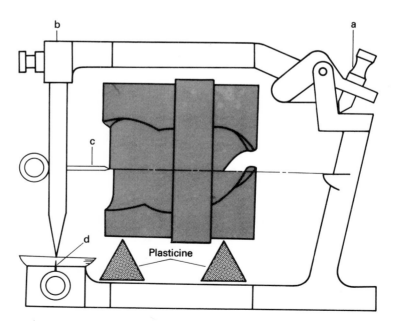

Fig. 4.8 Mounting casts on a fixed condylar angle articulator with the aid of Plasticine; a, lateral axis control arm; b, incisal guidance pin; c, incisal indicator pin; d, incisal guidance table.

cast placed on them (Fig. 4.8). The following adjustments are then carried out.

    a The junction of the centre line and the occlusal table should contact the apex of the incisal indicator pin (Fig. 4.8).
    b The occlusal surface of the upper occlusal rim should be aligned with an imaginery line, drawn from the apex of the incisal indicator pin to notches or a bar on the posterior pillars of the articulator. An elastic band circumscribing the notches and incisal indicator pin hole may be found helpful when aligning the occlusal rim.
    c The casts should be centrally positioned between the condylar axis.

5 The incisal indicator pin is removed and the upper arm of the articulator raised and stabilized in this position.
6 Plaster of Paris and water are mixed to a creamy consistency and a large increment placed on the base of the upper cast. The upper arm of the articulator is gently pressed into the mounting plaster, until the incisal guidance pin contacts the incisal table. More mounting plaster is added until it is flush with the top of the articulator arm. The mounting plaster is allowed to set.
7 After removal of the supporting Plasticine, the articulator is inverted by placing the top of the upper arm on the bench.
8 A further mix of plaster is made and the lower cast mounted in the manner described for the upper. It is important that the incisal guidance pin contacts the incisal table, since the pin maintains the vertical dimension throughout subsequent procedures.
9 The mounting plaster is trimmed, then smoothed with sandpaper and the articulator cleaned of plaster debris.

SIMPLE HINGE OR PLANE LINE ARTICULATOR

This articulator produces the simple opening and closing movements of the temporomandibular joint. Wear may take place at the hinge, introducing a lateral deflection. Some articulators incorporate means for adjustment to accommodate wear, and those devoid of this adjustment should be discarded once wear develops in the hinge.

1 The upper arm of the articulator should be parallel to the lower arm when the casts have been mounted (Fig. 4.9). The casts are trimmed to allow for this. Occasionally, it may be necessary to trim the posterior edge of the base of the upper cast to allow the upper arm of the articulator to be lowered.

2 The base of each cast is deeply scored, occlusal rims and casts sealed as described for mounting on an average value articulator the integral unit soaked in water.

3 The arms of the articulator are smeared lightly with petroleum jelly. Excess use of grease may cause the casts to fall off the articulator during subsequent procedures.

4 The vertical dimension adjusting screw at the rear of the articulator is adjusted to allow the upper arm to lie parallel to the lower arm.

5 Plaster is mixed to a creamy consistency and an increment placed on a flexible pad. The lower arm of the articulator is placed into the mounting plaster with its heel sitting on the pad, with plaster contacting the posterior localizing block (Fig. 4.9). More plaster is placed over the lower arm until there is sufficient to cover the base of the lower cast at a height of about 2 cm.

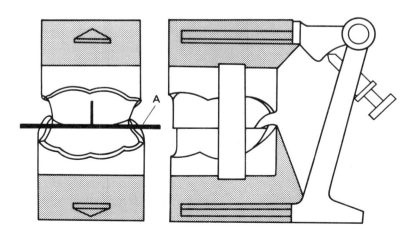

Fig. 4.9 Mounting casts on a plane line articulator with the aid of a T-shaped wire (A).

6   The upper arm of the articulator is raised and the base of the lower cast placed in the plaster mound. The following adjustments are then made.

   a   The occlusal plane should be equidistant from the arms of the articulator and parallel to the bench when viewed from every angle (Fig. 4.9).
   b   The centre line should be perpendicular (Fig. 4.9). Two pieces of wire soldered in the form of a letter T and attached to the occlusal rims as shown in Fig. 4.9 (A) may be helpful.
   c   The posterior border of the upper cast should approximate with the upper localizing block on the articulator (Fig. 4.9).
   d   The centre of the articulator should lie along the centre of the casts (Fig. 4.9).

7   The mounting plaster is smoothed to an outward taper by use of a plaster knife, then allowed to set.

8   A second mix of plaster is placed on the base of the upper cast, the upper arm of the articulator is inserted into the mounting plaster, followed by further additions to cover the arm completely. The mounting plaster is smoothed to produce a flat top with outward tapering sides.

9   The mounting plaster is allowed to set, then removed from the articulator to allow trimming on an electric trimmer. It is important that the walls of the casts are not reduced and that contact is maintained with the localizing blocks. The top of the upper is trimmed flat and parallel to the occlusal plane.

10 All plaster-work is smoothed with sandpaper and sharp edges are rounded slightly, then the plaster is coated with French chalk. The articulator is cleaned of plaster debris.

11 Finally, the vertical dimension adjustment screw is set. The locking nut is loosened and the adjustment screw rotated until its apex contacts the shoulder on the opposing arm of the articulator. The locking nut is tightened to prevent movement of the adjusting screw.

   An experienced operator usually mounts the upper and lower casts using one mix of plaster of Paris.

5 Partial Dentures

Diagnosis, treatment planning and any preliminary conservative treatment considered necessary is completed before considering the design of the denture.

STUDY CASTS

Upper and lower alginate impressions are taken for the construction of study casts (see Chapter 1). These are duplicated, one set is mounted on an articulator, whilst the second set is surveyed on a parallelometer. When correctly mounted on an articulator, they allow a thorough study of the occlusion from every angle, especially the lingual aspect which is not visible in the mouth. Any cuspal locking and occlusal paths are noted and where possible corrected by the dental surgeon.

COMPONENT PARTS

A partial denture may comprise the following components (Fig. 5.1).

Abutment. Any tooth in the natural dentition which is adjacent to a saddle or helps in the retention of, or support of a partial denture.

Saddle. That part of the denture which replaces lost alveolar tissue and normally contains the replacing teeth.

Support units. Means by which vertical occlusal load is transmitted to the alveolar bone, (a) through the saddle to the edentulous

63

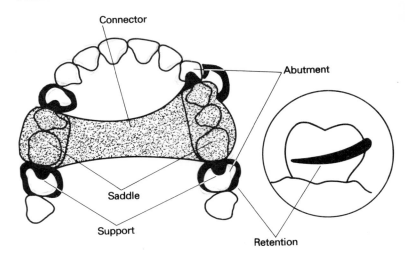

Fig. 5.1 Components of a partial denture.

alveolar bone; (b) through metallic extensions positioned on the natural dentition.

Retentive units. Means by which a partial denture is retained in the mouth. This is normally achieved by flexible metallic extensions encircling abutment teeth to enter undercut areas and called clasps.

Connector units. That part of the denture which combines components to form an integral unit.

Tagging. That part of a metallic structure used to form mechanical bonding with a non-metallic denture base.

PRINCIPLES OF DESIGN

The design of a partial denture is finalized through consultation between dentist and technician; the dentist discussing the clinical limitations, the technician raising the technical considerations. In general terms, the principles which should be followed are discussed below, but the process of designing need not necessarily follow the sequence laid out.

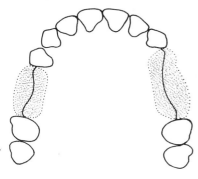

Fig. 5.2 Outline the saddle areas.

1.0 *Outline the saddle areas to be incorporated in the denture design* (Fig. 5.2).

The saddles to be incorporated in a design need not necessarily fill all the edentulous spaces present in the mouth.

1.1 A saddle is incorporated when tooth movement is envisaged. This may be drifting of adjacent teeth into the edentulous space or overeruption of teeth from the opposing dentition.

1.2 A saddle is omitted when tooth migration is unlikely and it is considered that appearance and mastication cannot be satisfactorily improved or restored. This decision is made only after full analysis of the occlusion from study casts mounted on an articulator.

1.3 A patient's psychological attitude to the appearance of the denture may be the sole criteria for incorporating a saddle.

2.0 *Classify the type of case according to the saddles to be incorporated.*

Many systems have been used to classify the partially dentate mouth. A simple and universally accepted classification is that formulated by Kennedy which is based on the edentulous areas being replaced by the denture. This has an advantage over other systems in that classification takes place before designing the component parts of the denture.

2.1 *Kennedy Class I.* The saddles are posterior to the standing teeth and are on both sides of the mouth. This is termed a bilateral free-end saddle (Fig. 5.3[1]).

Modifications. Additional saddles are termed modifications of the classification. Therefore, a Class I with one additional saddle is referred to as a Class I modification I (generally written as Mod. I). The modification number increases as the number of saddles increases.

2.2 *Kennedy Class II.* There is one saddle posterior to the standing teeth. It is termed a unilateral free-end saddle (Fig. 5.3[3]).

Modifications. Additional saddles which would not make the case a Class I are given a modification number.

2.3 *Kennedy Class III.* There is one saddle with the natural teeth standing anteriorly and posteriorly. It is termed a unilateral bounded saddle (Fig. 5.3[5]).

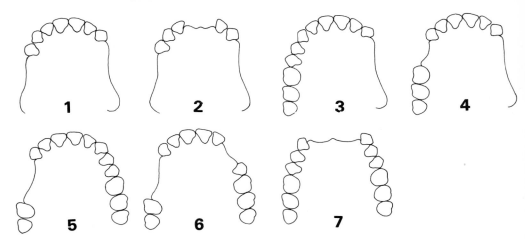

Fig. 5.3 Classify the type of case according to the saddle areas to be incorporated in the denture design: 1, Kennedy Class I; 2, Class I, Mod. I; 3, Kennedy Class II; 4, Class II, Mod. II; 5, Kennedy Class III; 6, Class III, Mod. I; 7, Kennedy Class IV.

Modifications. Additional saddles which would not classify the case as a Class I or Class II are given modification numbers.

2.4 *Kennedy Class IV*. The saddle is anterior of the natural dentition (Fig. 5.3[7]).

Modifications. There are no modifications of this classification because they would automatically place the case in one of the previous three categories.

The process of classification commences always with the class I and progresses through the classes until the case can be categorized.

3.0 *Classify the cast according to its load distribution.*

3.1 When the occlusal load is to be directed through metallic extensions to the standing teeth it is classified as being tooth-borne. The alveolar bone surrounding the natural dentition is said to be capable of absorbing greater occlusal loads than the bone in an edentulous area. Therefore, whenever possible, a denture should be tooth-supported.

3.2 When the occlusal load is to be directed through the saddles to the underlying alveolar bone it is classified as being mucosal or tissue-borne. A mucosal-borne denture is constructed as a temporary measure or when lengthy technical procedures associated with a tooth-borne denture are considered uneconomical.

3.3 When the occlusal load is to be distributed between edentulous alveolar bone and the standing teeth it is classified as a combination denture. This is necessary when few teeth are standing and the load is likely to be too great for the natural dentition, and in all free-end saddle cases.

4.0 *Make a preliminary choice of materials in which the denture is to be constructed.*

Decisions should be based upon a knowledge and understanding of the physical properties of the materials available, coupled with the estimated production costs. The reader is advised to study textbooks on dental materials to obtain the necessary information, but the principles of selection may be stated briefly.

4.1 The base may be constructed in acrylic resin when costs must be kept low. Most mucosal-borne dentures are constructed in this material.

4.2 The fitting surface of the saddle of a metal denture may be constructed in acrylic resin when additions, relining or alterations are envisaged.

4.3 Partial dentures made to a skeletal design should be constructed in cobalt chromium or a gold alloy. The type of alloy used depends upon the design features of the denture, the physical properties of the alloy and the production costs involved.

4.4 The final decision on which material to use may only be possible after costing and considering the various alternative designs.

5.0 *Plan the saddle support for a tooth-borne denture.*

This is accomplished by the use of rigid metallic extensions positioned on the standing teeth (Fig. 5.4).

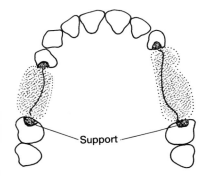

Fig. 5.4 Plan the saddle support for a tooth-borne denture.

a Occlusal rest. This extends into a prepared area on the occlusal surface of an abutment tooth (Fig. 5.5[1]).

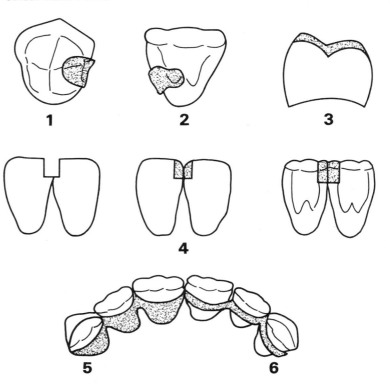

Fig. 5.5 Types of supporting units which may be incorporated in a partial denture.

b Onlay. This generally covers the whole of the occlusal surface of a tooth. Besides offering support it also corrects the occlusion (Fig. 5.5³).

c Cingulum rest. This extends into a prepared area on the cingulum of an anterior tooth (Fig. 5.5²).

d Embrasure hook. This normally extends into a prepared embrasure between two anterior teeth (Fig. 5.5⁴).

e Continuous clasp. This is a metal bar which embraces the cingulum of the anterior teeth (Fig. 5.5⁶).

f Lingual plate. This is a metal plate embracing much of the lingual aspect of anterior teeth (Fig. 5.5⁵) and generally the gingival tissues also.

5.1   Supporting teeth should be physiologically sound, with their

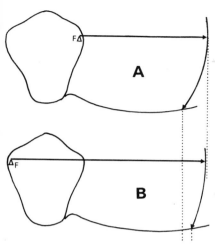

Fig. 5.6 Careful positioning of an occlusal rest (F) can distribute the load between tooth and tissue: A, high rotatory force; B, reduced rotatory force.

long axis at a right-angle to the alveolar bone. There is less possibility of tooth movement when occlusal forces are directed at 90° to the bone. It is recognized that this is not always possible.

5.2 Distribute the load over as many teeth as possible. A tooth is considered capable of supporting double its normal load. Therefore, as the length of a saddle increases so should the number of supporting teeth be increased. Anterior and posterior ends of a saddle should be supported whenever possible.

5.3 The load applied to a tooth may be decreased by moving the supporting unit to that part of the tooth furthest from the saddle area. This distributes the load to other abutment teeth or to the alveolar bone beneath a saddle.

5.4 Support for a Kennedy Class I and II classified dentures should be well anterior of the saddles. This has the effect of dividing the load between standing teeth and edentulous alveolar bone (Fig. 5.6). At the same time it produces a more vertical loading on the edentulous bone which minimizes bone resorption (Fig. 5.6).

5.5 Support is most effective when movement of the supporting teeth is prevented by contacting adjacent teeth.

5.6 Supporting units should be placed on both sides of an isolated tooth to prevent its rotation.

5.7 Supporting units should not interfere with the articulation or occlusion. An imbalance of the occlusal table may result in pain in the temporomandibular joint.

6.0 *Survey the study cast.*
This is covered in detail in Chapter 2, it will suffice to summarize the process.

6.1 Determine the path of insertion of the denture.

6.2 Determine usable tooth and tissue undercuts and their depth.

6.3 Determine the presence of unusable undercuts.

6.4 Eliminate unusable undercuts.

7.0 *Classify the survey line according to Blatterfein.*
Blatterfein classified survey lines according to their position on the tooth. The area of a tooth nearest to a saddle he referred to as the near zone and that furthest from the saddle, the far zone.

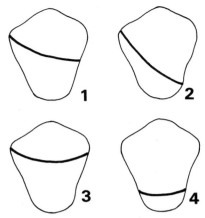

Fig. 5.7 Classify the survey line. Illustration shows Blatterfein's classification: 1, medium; 2, diagonal; 3, high; 4, low.

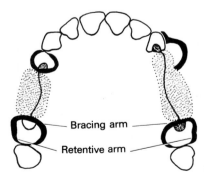

Fig. 5.8 Plan flexible retentive and rigid bracing units.

a Medium survey line. Although situated approximately across the centre of a tooth it exhibits a slight occlusogingival incline from the near to the far zone. (Fig. 5.7).
b Diagonal survey line. This travels diagonally from near the occlusal surface in the near zone to near the gingiva in the far zone (Fig. 5.7).
c High survey line. This is found near the occlusal surface of a tooth, often being parallel to the gingival margin (Fig. 5.7).
d Low survey line. This is situated close to and may be parallel to the gingival margin of a tooth (Fig. 5.7).

8.0 *Plan flexible retentive and rigid bracing units* (Fig. 5.8).
These units are generally named clasps. A clasp arm may consist of two portions: a retentive portion which is thin and flexible and rests in an undercut area on an abutment tooth (Fig. 5.9); a thicker bracing portion which rests on or above the bulbous area of a tooth and transmits lateral loads to the natural dentition (Fig. 5.9). The various types of clasp are illustrated in Figs. 5.10 and 5.11.
8.1 Clasps may be placed in one of two groups:

a Occlusally approaching. This is when the retentive arm approaches the tooth undercut from an occlusal direction (Fig. 5.9).
b Gingivally approaching. This is a clasp which approaches the tooth undercut from a gingival direction (Fig. 5.11). Such clasps produce a trip action when being forced out of an undercut. This action is said to be the most effective means of retaining a denture, but the clasp arm may be difficult to design from the point of view of patient comfort. Consequently, occlusally approaching clasps are often preferred, although perhaps less effective as a retainer, and sometimes more conspicuous than a gingivally approaching clasp.

8.2 The retentive portion of a clasp arm should be sufficiently flexible to allow it to enter and to be removed from a tooth undercut. This is dependent upon the design of the arm and upon the alloy used in its construction.
8.3 The bracing portion of a clasp arm should be rigid. A lateral

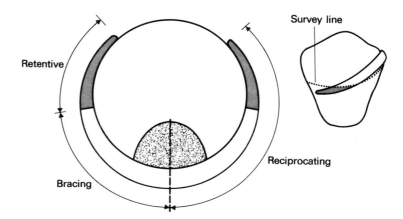

Fig. 5.9 Component portions of a clasp. This illustrates an occlusally approaching clasp.

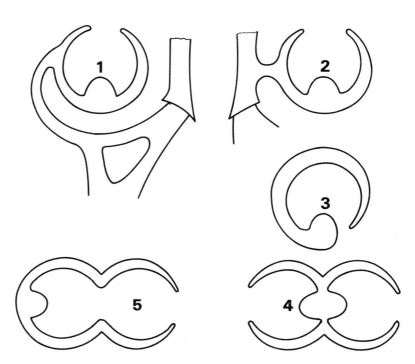

Fig. 5.10 Types of occlusally approaching clasp. All the following may also be called circumferential clasps: 1, reverse back action clasp; 2, back action clasp; 3, ring clasp; 4, embrasure clasp; 5, extended arm clasp.

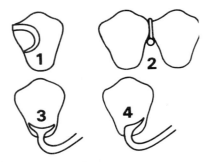

Fig. 5.11 Other types of clasp. Occlusally approaching: 1, Recurved arm clasp; 2, ball clasp or Rusch anchor. Gingivally approaching or bar clasps; 3, Roach T; 4, Roach L.

load is best transmitted to a tooth through a rigid bracing portion of a clasp arm. Its rigidity depends upon the design and alloy used.

8.4 Clasp arms should be inconspicuous when in the mouth.

8.5 A clasp should not increase the width of the occlusal table or interfere with the occlusion because it would have the effect of increasing the occlusal load on a tooth.

8.6 Every retentive clasp arm should be accompanied by another clasp on the opposite side of the tooth (Fig. 5.9). This opposes the displacing force exerted on an abutment tooth from a retentive clasp arm each time the denture is inserted or removed from the mouth. Such forces could eventually lead to loosening of the tooth, unless opposed by a clasp arm, continuous clasp or lingual plate. The opposing clasp arm is termed a reciprocating clasp.

8.7 All clasp arms should be so designed as to maintain the mouth in a healthy condition and avoid causing caries or physiological changes in the gingiva.

9.0 *Plan additional support and retention.*

Clasps are most effective when the displacing forces acting on a denture are transmitted in a vertical occlusal direction. When rotatory forces act about a supporting unit, the retentive portion of a clasp arm may move gingivally and not contact the tooth. This effect may be minimized by the use of auxiliary supports which indirectly help to retain the denture by preventing rotation, and are termed indirect retainers. The various types of indirect retainer are additional occlusal rests, continuous clasp, lingual plate, palatal arms and embrasure hooks.

9.1 Indirect retainers should be rigid.

9.2 They should prevent rotation of the denture.

9.3 They should not interfere with the articulation or occlusion.

9.4 They should be so shaped as to be readily tolerated by the patient.

9.5 Their effectiveness increases the further they are placed from a rotating point (the fulcrum point).

10.0 *Position and shape of connectors.*

Connectors are divided into two groups:

a Major connector. This is the main connector which joins the saddles and to which all other components are attached (Fig. 5.12).

b Minor connector. This joins components to the major connector.

10.1 All connectors must be rigid.

10.2 All connectors should be so designed as to be readily tolerated by the patient.

10.3 Major connectors should be a minimum of 4 mm from the gingival margin of standing teeth to prevent trauma to the tissue (Fig. 5.13). When this is impossible to achieve, the gingival margin is relieved and the connector continued on to the lingual or palatal surface of the tooth up to the survey line, to completely cover the

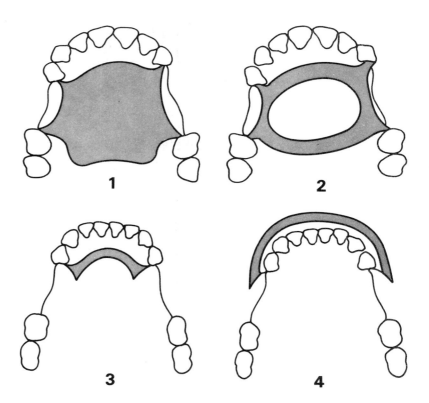

Fig. 5.12 Types of major connector: 1, palatal plate; 2, anterior and posterior palatal bars; 3, lingual bar; 4, buccal bar.

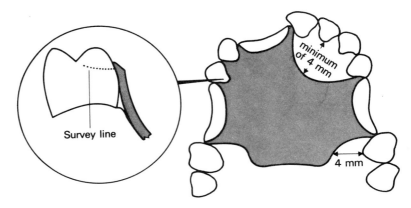

Fig. 5.13 Major connectors should be a minimum of 4 mm from the gingival margins of standing teeth or alternatively cover the gingiva and terminate above the survey line on the tooth.

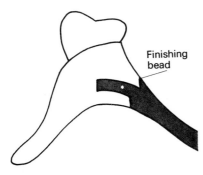

Fig. 5.14 The border of a metal major connector with an acrylic resin saddle is termed a finishing bead.

gingiva (Fig. 5.13). This also prevents the formation of a stagnation area between connector and clasp.

10.4 Major connectors must be rigidly attached to saddles, at which point it should widen to produce a border called a finishing bead (Fig. 5.14). A finishing bead is so shaped as to prevent percolation of mouth fluids between the major connector and an acrylic resin saddle.

10.5 A slight rotation of a major connector during function should not result in trauma of the tissues. This especially applies to a lingual bar incorporated in a Kennedy Class I bilateral free-end saddle (Fig. 5.15).

10.6 A major connector should be clear of muscle attachments by 2–4 mm. This especially applies to a lingual bar in relation to a lingual fraenum (Fig. 5.15).

10.7 A minor connector should cross the gingival margin at 90°, and the gingiva relieved to prevent trauma.

10.8 A minor connector should be placed in an interstitial area, the deepest part of which should be relieved, and so shaped as to blend into this area. It should have thickness by its penetration into the interstitial area whilst its mesiodistal width should be narrow (Fig. 5.16).

10.9 A minor connector should meet a major connector at a right-angle and flare at the joint (Fig. 5.16). This increases the strength of the joint, and prevents the formation of a stagnant angle.

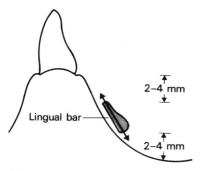

Fig. 5.15 A lingual bar should be well clear of muscle attachments and gingival margins and be parallel to the alveolar process.

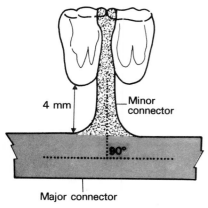

Fig. 5.16 A minor connector should be placed in an interstitial area and be at 90° to the major connector.

10.10 When a minor connector joins a component to a saddle (such as joining a clasp to a saddle) it should be as thin as possible, compatible with strength, so as not to interfere with the area available for the denture teeth.

11.0 *Form a peripheral seal.*
The physical retentive forces of adhesion, cohesion and atmospheric pressure are more efficient when a seal exists around the periphery of a denture. The seal is achieved in an upper denture by scribing a shallow groove into the cast to thicken the periphery of the denture. This causes the denture to sink slightly into the oral tissue to form a seal. It should follow the outline of the denture from saddle area to saddle area, be D-shaped, no deeper than 0·5 mm and no wider than 1·0 mm. The groove is not cut into the periphery of a labial or buccal saddle area.

11.1 Finish the border of a denture behind prominent rugae, so that it becomes unnoticeable to the patient's tongue.

11.2 Never scribe a peripheral groove into rugae because this may cause the rugae to swell and become inflamed.

11.3 Never continue a peripheral groove on to the gingival tissues. This may cause the gingiva to swell and eventually result in the tissue receding from the cervical margin of a tooth.

12.0 *Transfer the design features to a draft prescription form.*
A number of designs may be possible for any one patient. Each should be noted on a draft prescription form and the technical procedures costed. It is then possible for the dentist to discuss the various designs and costings with the patient. Finally, the designs are assessed against clinical limitations and a design agreed. This is transferred to a laboratory prescription form with other relevant information.

6 The Pattern

Once a denture has been designed, the master cast is duplicated in an investment material. This is a material containing silicon dioxide (a heat-resistant material called a refractory) its particles being held together by plaster of Paris when a gold alloy is to be used, and a phosphate (ammonium diacid phosphate) when a cobalt chromium alloy is to be cast. The structure is formed in wax or plastic on an investment cast and the whole embedded in more investment material. This is heated to melt the wax, thereby forming a mould, and molten metal is poured into it. The procedure is termed 'the lost wax process' and has been in use since ancient times.

The wax structure is called the pattern and the best results are obtained by the use of special waxes which burn readily and leave no residue in the mould at casting temperatures. These casting waxes are obtainable in sheet form of various thicknesses, in the shape of a clasp or as rods of different shapes and thicknesses.

One method of forming the pattern is to commence with the saddles, followed by the support units, clasping, major connectors, minor connectors and finally the junctions of the units smoothed. The thickness of wax used depends upon the alloy, the physical properties required of the finished denture and the experience of the operator. The measurements given in this chapter are average and acceptable for beginners, allowing for slight thinning of wax and for a lack of experience at casting metal into a mould. They are modified with experience.

SADDLES

Without relief

1 The outline of the denture is drawn on the investment cast.

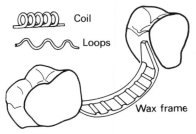

Fig. 6.1 Types of retentive form for attaching an acrylic resin saddle to a metal structure.

2 A piece of 0·6 mm casting wax is cut, sufficient to cover the saddle area. This is softened slightly by holding above a Bunsen burner flame (softening is often unnecessary in warm weather, the wax being quite soft and pliable), then adapted closely to the saddle area, care being taken not to reduce the thickness of the wax. It should be at least 2 mm larger than the outline drawn on the cast and cover the proximal surface of the abutment teeth. This wax is trimmed to shape using a Le Cron or Ash No. 5 wax carver. It should finish about 2 mm over the crest of the ridge on the labial or buccal aspect, about 2 mm past the gingival margins of the standing teeth on the palatal aspect, and 2 mm short of the marginal ridge of the abutment teeth to form a cone-shape on the proximal surface (Fig. 6.1). It is sealed to the investment cast by warming the blade of a wax carver and running it along the edge of the wax. Care is taken to prevent wax flowing over a large area of the cast, which may result in a lengthy finishing procedure.

3 Mechanical means of attaching an acrylic resin denture base material to the metal saddle must be incorporated in the design. This is achieved by forming loops or a coil in wax which is sealed to the saddle and termed tagging (Fig. 6.1). The loops or coil must not interfere with the positioning of the denture teeth. A coil may be formed out of 0·8 mm wax rod by bending it around a piece of 1 mm wire. The base of each loop is sealed to the saddle with wax, the ends being sealed to the proximal extensions of the saddle to form a rigid unit.

With relief

This is used when acrylic resin is to contact the tissue in the saddle area. The metal structure is formed in a lattice design forming tagging to allow the resin to interlock with the metal.

1 A piece of 0·6 mm sheet casting wax is cut into a triangular shape, the size of the outline drawn on the proximal surface of the abutment teeth and sealed to this area of the cast (Fig. 6.1).

2 Preformed lattice-designed wax is available from which the tagging may be formed. A piece is cut and adapted to the outline drawn on the cast. It terminates at and is sealed to the proximal triangle of wax on the abutment teeth and its buccal or labial periphery sealed to the cast (Fig. 6.1).

3   Alternatively, 1·15×1·75 mm D-shaped or round wax may be formed into a lattice or ladder design (Fig. 6.1) and attached to the proximal triangle of wax on the abutment teeth. The tagging is placed just lingual or palatal to the ridge when it is envisaged that a problem may be encountered with positioning of denture teeth. Wax is extended posteriorly on to the unrelieved area of the cast in the case of a free-end saddle. This supports the substructure during later stages of denture construction.

SUPPORT

It is normal practice for the dentist to prepare teeth to accept support units (Fig. 6.2). This section of the pattern should therefore reconstruct the original shape of the tooth, be sufficiently rigid and strong, yet not interfere with occlusal relationships. Their formation requires a wax which is hard and easily carvable, without chipping. Wax used in the formation of inlays (inlay wax) is ideal. Molten wax is applied to the required area in a controlled manner.

The blade of a wax carver is warmed in a Bunsen burner flame and a small increment of inlay wax melted on it. The carver is returned to the flame, this time ensuring the neck and not the tip of

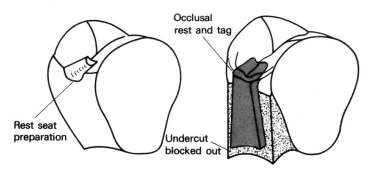

Fig. 6.2 An occlusal rest and tag.

the blade is heated. This causes the wax to travel away from the heat source which results in the wax remaining at the tip of the blade where it is required. By careful control of the temperature, it is possible to place the wax against the appropriate area of the cast and by using the carver in the manner of a pen to draw the required shape in wax. Such a method prevents indiscriminate coverage of the cast with wax, which would result in a lengthy finishing technique. The occlusion should be checked throughout the procedure. Occlusal carving may be achieved by gently heating the blade of a Le Cron carver and lightly pressing it on the surface of the wax. It will be found that the rounded contour of the blade readily produces the side of a cusp and the marginal ridge simultaneously.

Occlusal rests

1   Occlusal rests should taper towards the centre of the tooth.
2   Where possible they should recontour the shape of the tooth, especially in the marginal ridge area (Fig. 6.2).
3   They should have sufficient thickness to produce a rigid unit (Fig. 6.2).
4   They should not interfere with the occlusion.

Onlays

1   Onlays should produce a smaller occlusal surface than exists on the natural tooth (Fig. 6.3).
2   The curvature of the outer walls should be a continuation of the curvature of the tooth (Fig. 6.3).
3   The top of cusps should be given a natural contour with no sharp areas (Fig. 6.3).
4   The occlusal carving should be kept shallow to reduce occlusal load.

Embrasure hooks

1   Embrasure hooks should recontour the prepared tooth.
2   They should have slightly rounded outer edges to reflect light in

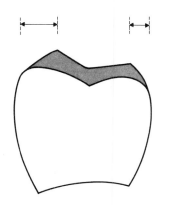

Fig. 6.3   The occlusal surface of an occlusal onlay should be narrower than the natural tooth.

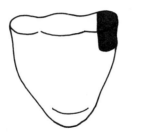

Fig. 6.4   An embrasure hook.

various directions and thereby be less conspicious in the mouth (Fig. 6.4).

RETENTION

Preformed patterns of clasps are obtainable, and they often do not require trimming once adapted to a cast. Many contain an occlusal rest portion which occasionally is too thin and so requires thickening. Better results are obtained by removing the rest portion and forming the rest in the manner described above. When preformed patterns are not available, D-shaped profile wax (1·15 mm×1·75 mm) may be used.

Occlusally approaching clasps

Circumferential clasp

The rest portion is removed from a preformed pattern and the occlusal rest formed in inlay wax.

1   The tapered end of the clasp is placed in the undercut area as denoted by the ledge on the tooth. The index finger of one hand is used to hold the clasp in position whilst the remainder of the clasp is adapted to the tooth. It is important that the lower edge of the clasp rests on the prepared ledge. The bracing arm is trimmed to length and tapered towards its tip. A similar method is adopted when using D-shaped profile wax, but both clasp arms must be tapered towards their tips (Fig. 6.5).

2   It is advisable to seal the pattern to the cast. This requires very careful temperature control of the wax carver blade. Carding wax may be used as the sealant because it has a lower melting point than pattern wax and it flows easily. It is also very soft and so may be trimmed with ease without damage to the pattern.

3   The clasp is sealed to the rest unit and the triangular proximal wax, which then becomes a minor connector, connecting the clasping unit to the saddle or tagging. The joint between rest, clasp and

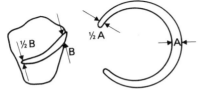

Fig. 6.5   The retentive portion of a clasp should be half the thickness of the bracing portion.

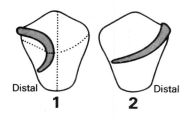

Fig. 6.6 Views of a recurved arm clasp: 1, buccal; 2, palatal.

minor connector will encroach on the space available for denture teeth, but this encroachment must be minimal.

Ring clasp

The waxing technique described above is used to form a ring clasp. The length of a ring clasp demands greater rigidity in the bracing portion than is required of a circumferential clasp. It is thickened with wax until about one-third thicker than its original dimensions.

Recurved arm clasp

This clasp is best confined to large teeth, otherwise it may be found difficult to construct and unsightly when in the mouth.
1 The retentive end of the clasp is bent around the shaft of a wax carver to form a C-shape (Fig. 6.6).
2 The tip of the clasp is placed in the undercut, and the curvature adjusted to bring the leading edge distal to the centre of the tooth with the remainder of the arm above the bulbous portion (Fig. 6.6). The length and shape of the bracing arm is adjusted and sealed to the cast.

Gingivally approaching clasps

These clasps consist of a bar with a retentive end in the shape of a letter L, T, or V. The bar emerges from the saddle and gently curves until it approaches the tooth along its long axis (Fig. 6.7). The bar may be slightly flared to produce a finishing bead at the periphery of the acrylic resin (Fig. 6.7). Care is taken to ensure that the bar does not interfere with the cheek or muscle attachments.

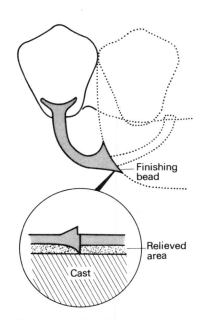

Fig. 6.7 A finishing bead may be formed at the junction of a bar clasp with an acrylic resin saddle.

Continuous clasps

This clasp has been superseded in the main by the lingual plate which is less bulky and more easily tolerated by the patient.
1 A strip of 0·2 mm sheet casting wax is cut and adapted to the cingulum area of the cast.

2   A length of round or D-shaped profile wax is adapted over the sheet wax and sealed to it with carding wax. This is carved to produce a pear-shape to resemble a thickened cingulum, the thickest area being towards the gingival area. Excess sheet wax is trimmed to allow the clasp to blend into the contour of the teeth. The distal extremities of a continuous clasp may terminate in retentive clasping units and embrasure hooks may also be incorporated in the design.

CONNECTORS

The strength of the denture relies upon the strength and rigidity of the connector which should be sufficiently thick to be rigid, yet be so shaped as to be well tolerated by the patient.

Major connectors

Lingual bar

A lingual bar should be pear-shaped where ever possible, because this shape is well tolerated by patients, but D-shaped bars may be used as an alternative.

1   A length of shaped profile wax is cut and adapted to the cast. It should follow the curvature of the gingival area of the standing teeth, but be at least 4 mm away from them. It should also be clear of the floor of the cast (Fig. 5.15). Long bars may be adapted in two pieces with a 1 mm space between them in the midline region. The space is filled with carding wax to seal the ends together and to the cast.

2   The bar is finished at the edge of the saddle which in some cases is denoted by the edge of the relieved area. A finishing bead is formed at the junction of the bar and saddle. A piece of D-shaped wax is placed on its side with its flat surface facing distally (Fig. 6.8). It is adapted to the border of the saddle, one end rising along the lingual edge of the triangular proximal saddle wax, and the other end curving distally towards the floor of the cast. Its mesial edge

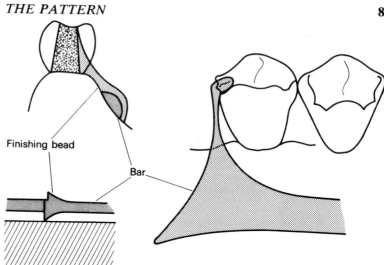

Fig. 6.8 Formation of a finishing bead between a lingual bar and acrylic resin saddle.

only is sealed to the cast by use of carding wax. The lingual bar is flared into the finishing bead by further use of wax. The finishing bead is chamfered to a thin section towards the occlusal surface of the abutment tooth, gradually increasing in thickness towards the bar until about 0·5 mm thicker than the bar. It is also chamfered to a thin section towards the floor of the cast. This produces a gradual rise towards the centre of the lingual bar.

Lingual plate

A lingual plate is a thin metallic base, covering the gingival tissue and formed to the lingual or palatal aspect of teeth. It may act as a bracing unit opposing a retentive clasp arm, it may cover small areas between a major connector and clasp arm to prevent the formation of a stagnation area, or it may act as a continuous plate to become an indirect retainer.

Short lingual plate

A short lingual plate requires a finished thickness of about 0·6 mm which demands a pattern thickness of around 0·65 mm.

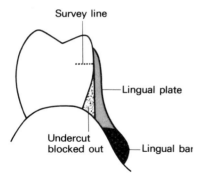

Fig. 6.9 Formation of a short lingual plate.

1 Depressions around standing teeth are flushed smooth with carding wax.

2 A piece of 0·65 mm sheet casting wax is adapted to the desired area to blend into the finishing bead and major connector but not to increase its thickness (Fig. 6.9). The occlusal edge of the plate should finish above the survey line whilst the mesial edge should blend into the shape of the proximal surface of the standing tooth (Fig. 6.9), but should not extend interstitially, where it could form an area which would be difficult to clean.

Continuous lingual plate

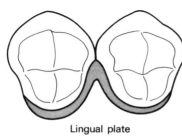

The continuous lingual plate covers the gingival tissue and rests on and conforms to the cingulum of anterior teeth. It is used in preference to a continuous clasp. The incisal limits should not be visible in the mouth (Fig. 6.10).

1 The upper limit of the plate and lower limit of the bar are outlined on the cast and the interstitial and gingival depressions smoothed with wax.

2 Pear-shaped profile wax is adapted along the lower border of the plate, trimmed to the saddles and sealed to the cast.

3 A strip of 0·65 mm sheet casting wax is adapted to the teeth with its lower limit resting on the lingual bar. It is trimmed to shape and sealed to cast and bar, and then blended into the shape of the bar (Fig. 6.10).

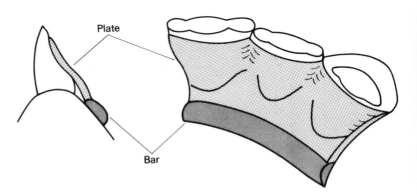

Fig. 6.10 A continuous lingual plate attached to a lingual bar.

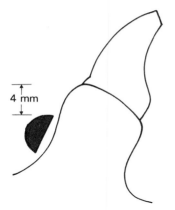

4 mm

Fig. 6.11 Position of a buccal bar.

Buccal bar

The method of adapting a bar to the buccal region of a cast is the same as for a lingual bar. It is placed as near the buccal sulcus as possible, yet clear of muscle attachments. Buccal bars are thinner but wider than the lingual bar. They are not readily tolerated by patients and, therefore, are confined to cases of extensive lingual inclination of anterior teeth (Fig. 6.11).

Palatal connectors

Palatal connectors may be narrow and thick and referred to as a bar, or wide and thin when it then becomes a plate. The thickness of a connector depends upon its width as Table 6.1 indicates.

Table 6.1 Dimensions of major connectors.

Width (mm)	Thickness (mm)	Form of wax profile
2	1·5	Bar
2–5	1·25	Bar
5–8	1·00	Sheet in two thicknesses 0·4 mm plus 0·6 mm
8–12	0·8	Sheet in two thicknesses 0·3 mm plus 0·5 mm
12 and above	Gradual decrease to 0·5 mm for full palatal coverage	Sheet in two thicknesses 0·2 mm plus 0·3 mm

These measurements may be increased according to the gold alloy being used or decreased by experienced operators when cobalt–chrome alloys are to be used. It will be seen from Table 6.1 that a pattern of a connector with a width above 5 mm can be adapted to the cast in two thicknesses of wax, but many technicians use one only.

1   A strip of the thinner wax is adapted to the cast, care being

taken to prevent thinning or damage to the wax. It is best adapted in two halves to prevent thinning, one on each side of the midline. This wax is trimmed 2 mm short of the peripheral groove and its edges sealed and carved to blend into the cast. The saddle may be formed out of the same piece of wax or the connector terminated at the edge of the saddle.

2   A length of triangular or D-shaped profile wax is adapted to form a finishing bead with the saddle, its flat surface being perpendicular and facing the palate (Fig. 6.12[1]). The finishing bead should taper to a thin section as it rises towards the occlusal surface along the mesioproximal or distoproximal corner of abutment teeth.

3   The second layer of wax is adapted over the first. It is trimmed to the edge of the peripheral groove and the top edge of the D-shaped finishing bead sealed to the cast (Fig. 6.12).

4   Alternatively, the profile wax may be omitted and the finishing bead formed by the edge of the second layer of sheet wax. Its edge should be sealed, then trimmed perpendicular (Fig. 6.12[2]). The interstitial embrasure between the denture and abutment tooth should be kept as wide as possible to prevent food being trapped in this area.

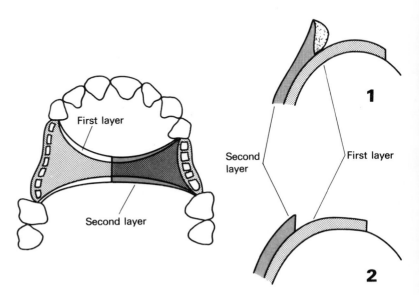

Fig. 6.12   A palatal plate may be formed in two layers, the second layer terminating in a finishing bead.

First layer

Second layer

Second layer

First layer

1

2

Minor connector

Some minor connectors are best adapted to the cast before the major connector.

1 When it is directly joined into a saddle.

2 When it is to be indistinguishable from the major connector, for example, when it is to be covered by the major connector. This produces a smooth surface to a casting, and the increased thickness imparts strength.

   Alternatively, the denture design may require the minor connector to be adapted upon completion of the major connector and D-shaped profile wax is used in these instances. The position of the connector will have been selected during the design stage. Normally, the profile wax is adapted to the interstitial area of the cast. It is kept at 90° to the major connector and covers the minimum gingival tissue, compatible with strength. It is sealed to the cast and component units with carding wax and carved to blend into each unit so as to eliminate sharp angles (Fig. 6.13).

Plastic patterns

Pliable plastic patterns may be used in preference to wax. They are sealed to the investment cast by use of an adhesive. It is essential for the adhesive to be thin and to cover the area of the profile only, otherwise molten metal will flow into the area originally occupied by the adhesive to result in a lengthy finishing procedure. Plastic components are joined by wax.

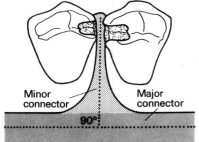

Fig. 6.13 The join between minor and major connectors is curved to eliminate sharp angles and prevent a stagnant area.

Full plates

The methods so far described have dealt with partial dentures only but the palate of a full denture may also be cast in metal.

1 When the master cast has been prepared with a relieved saddle area, preformed wax mesh or loops should be adapted to the cast. It can be helpful for later stages, if the position of the denture teeth can be visualized and the tagging adapted so as not to interfere with their position (Fig. 6.14). Tagging should not traverse the crest of the ridge in the anterior region but may traverse the posterior ridge by about 2 mm. The saddle is terminated at the palatal border of the relieved area.

2   The finished thickness of a gold full palate should be around 0·8 mm, although experienced operators can produce thinner castings. It is adapted in two thicknesses of wax, 0·35 mm and 0·5 mm, which allows 0·05 mm for possible thinning of the wax during adaption

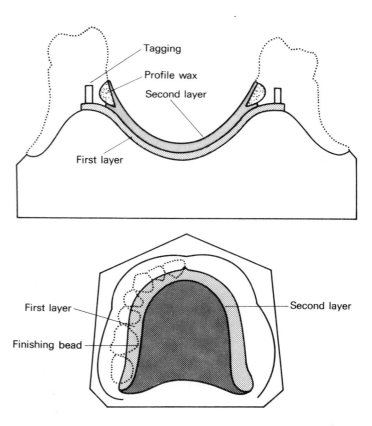

Fig. 6.14   Forming a full plate. The position of denture teeth must be visualized when positioning the finishing bead and tagging.

and for loss of metal during the finishing process. Beginners are advised to adapt each thickness of wax in two halves to reduce the possibility of thinning, and join them in the centre of the palate by the use of carding wax. They are normally sufficiently soft and pliable for use without heating during the summer months, but may be softened over a Bunsen burner flame in cold weather. The thinnest wax is the first to be adapted. It may be continued into the saddle area to form tagging, or terminated at previously adapted tagging (Fig. 6.14). It is trimmed short of the peripheral groove and its edge chamfered.

3   A finishing bead is formed at the required junction between saddle area and palate. Triangular or D-shaped profile wax is used. Its edge placed on the cast with a flat surface facing the palate, the rounded portion of a D-shaped profile facing the saddle. About 10 mm of the profile is extended past the posterior border of the pattern and waxed to the cast. It is then adapted to an even curvature over the previously laid sheet wax. The finished denture needs to be visualized and the beading so positioned as to form a natural progression from palate to teeth. When the saddle has been relieved the flat surface of the D-shaped profile should conform to the palatal aspect of the raised relief. The posterior extensions are then curved to finish behind the tuberosities to form the posterior extremity of the denture (Fig. 6.14). It is sealed on the palatal surface with carding wax and carved to form a smooth contour.

4   The thicker sheet of wax is also adapted to the cast in two pieces, trimmed to terminate at the posterior edge of the post dam and half-way up the bead, then sealed down. It is carved to blend into the beading.

5   Alternatively, the bead may be omitted and the periphery of the second sheet wax used as the finishing bead.

6   A metal saddle which does not have its undersurface relieved will require the use of tagging in the form of loops, coil or spikes with a rail. They may be placed over the crest of the ridge in the posterior region and fractionally palatal to the crest of the ridge in the anterior region. What is important is that they should not interfere with the positioning of denture teeth.

Finishing the pattern

A smooth pattern produces a smooth casting and reduces finishing time. Various commercial products are available for the purpose of smoothing the wax which also lower its surface tension; a desirable property when investing. A cheap and effective method is to use a liquid detergent such as Teepol.

A pledget of cotton wool is wrapped around the end of a bur, soaked in Teepol and the excess squeezed out. It is warmed over a Bunsen burner flame, then rubbed over the pattern. The process is repeated until the whole pattern is smooth and ready for the next stage which is the attachment of sprue formers.

SPRUEING

Although the pattern forms a mould inside the refractory material, some means must be available for pouring molten metal into the mould (Fig. 6.15). This requires the formation of a cone-shaped funnel and a passage from the funnel to the mould. These are best formed at the time of embedding the pattern. The funnel is termed a crucible and may be formed by the use of wax, plastic or metal either at the time of pouring the refractory cast or during the embedding procedure. Wax, plastic or metal rods are used to form the passage and are called sprue formers.

Point of attachment of the sprue former

The essence of sprueing is to ensure continuous flow of metal into the mould. The walls of a mould can assist or impede the flow, depending upon the position of the sprue, or the thickness of the pattern at the point of attachment. Since the design variations of a partial denture can be great, it is possible only to state guidelines to follow with regard to the point of attachment of sprue formers.

1   Maximum impedance to flow occurs when the sprue former makes an angle of 90° to the pattern (Fig. 6.16).

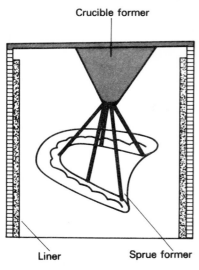

Crucible former

Liner   Sprue former

Fig. 6.15 A pattern within a casting cylinder.

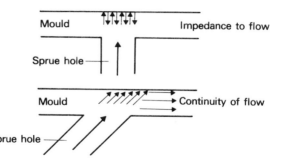

Fig. 6.16 Maximum impedance to flow occurs when a sprue former makes an angle of 90° to the pattern.

2 Always consider the crucible, sprue hole and mould as being a wedge, the crucible being the thickest section. There should be a gradual decrease in thickness throughout (Fig. 6.17). Therefore, a thick section of pattern should lead to a thin section and never the other way around.

3 It is better to use too many sprue formers than to have too few, which may result in a miscast.

4 All sprue formers should approach the pattern from the same direction. This minimizes the possibility of turbulence as the metal converges in the mould.

5 Sprue formers should be so arranged that the mould trails behind the direction of movement of the centrifugal casting machine (Fig. 6.18). This allows the casting force to thrust the metal into the mould and exert pressure on the metal until solidification is complete. Such castings have a high density and low porosity.

6 Sprue formers should be so positioned as to facilitate removal of the sprues from the cast metal denture base.

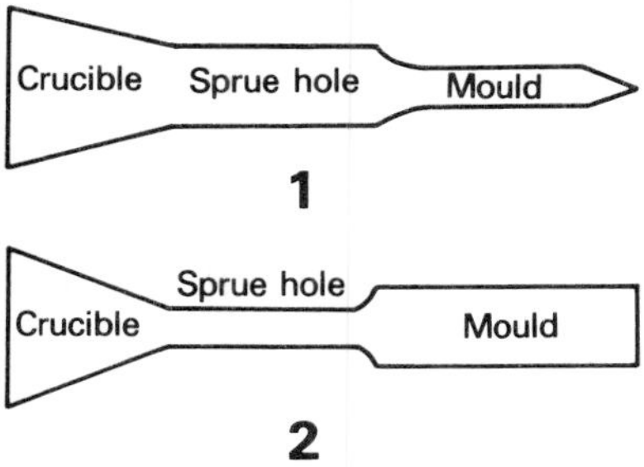

Diameter

The sprue former should be thicker than the pattern to which it is attached, because as metal solidifies it contracts, and draws molten metal from adjacent thicker sections. Since the thin sections solidify and contract first, they will draw molten metal from thicker sections which in turn require metal on which to draw. Sprues may act as ideal reservoirs for these thicker sections. Failure to cater for this

Fig. 6.17 The crucible, sprue hole and mould should be considered as being a wedge-shape: 1, correct; 2, incorrect.

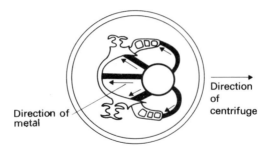

Fig. 6.18 Sprue formers should be so arranged that centrifugal force thrusts the metal into the mould.

may result in a reduction in density of the casting by the presence of voids called porosity. Porosity is also reduced by a slight narrowing of the thick sprue former at the point of attachment with the pattern (Fig. 6.19).

A slight problem arises when steam pressure is used to force metal into the mould. The alloy is melted in the crucible at the head of the sprue holes. The surface tension forces within the molten alloy prevent the alloy entering the sprue holes during the melting stage. When a sprue hole is large, the weight of the metal may be greater than the surface tension forces which results in the alloy trickling down the sprue holes to produce a gravity cast. Such castings are normally porous. This may be prevented by use of sprue formers no greater in thickness than 2 mm, with the lack of bulk being compensated for by thickening the sprue former at a point 2 mm from the pattern (Fig. 6.19), to form a reservoir thicker than the pattern.

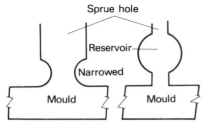

Fig. 6.19 Narrowing of a sprue former may reduce porosity, as may a reservoir on a thin sprue former.

Length

The length of a sprue hole, coupled with its diameter, affects the speed at which metal enters the mould. Every mould contains gases which are expelled ahead of the in-flowing metal. The length of sprue hole should therefore be adjusted to allow the mould gases to escape through the investment mould, yet also allow the mould to be filled before the metal solidifies. The rate of expulsion of mould gases is also dependent upon the permeability of the investment material, the thickness of the material between the pattern and the outside atmosphere (the back-up investment), and the presence of gas vents. Ideally, there should be no more than 1 cm of embedding investment surrounding an investment cast, and sprue holes should be no longer than 2 cm. It may be necessary to increase the length of subsidiary sprue holes which feed remote areas of the mould, but they should be kept to a minimum length.

Attaching the sprue former

The method of attaching sprue formers differs slightly depending upon the location of the crucible former, which may be in the base of the cast or suspended above the pattern.

Sprueing when the crucible former is cast-located

1   A length of 5·0 mm round profile wax is adapted to the floor of the cast from the crucible hole to the lower edge of the pattern (Fig. 6.20¹). It is sealed to the cast and pattern, leaving no space between the sprue former and cast. These are termed primary sprue formers and are attached to the major connector.

2   Secondary sprue formers are made from 2·5 mm thickness of round wax profile and are attached to thick areas remote from the major connector. They may be lifted off the floor of the cast and given a gentle curve from the crucible hole to the pattern. They should approach the pattern from the same direction as the primary sprue former (Fig. 6.20¹) and be kept as short as possible.

3   A wax extension, about 5 mm in height and the diameter of the crucible hole, is formed and sealed over the hole and to the sprue formers. The crucible is filled with wax to raise the base of the cast by 5 mm (Fig. 6.20¹). Alternatively, the cast may be placed on and sealed to a plastic crucible former. This has an extension which projects through the crucible hole, to which the sprue formers are waxed (Fig. 6.20²).

Sprueing when the crucible former is suspended

1   A hollow cone is formed from modelling wax by wrapping it

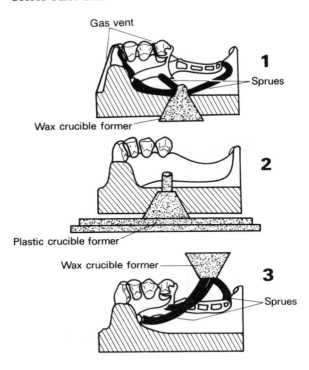

Fig. 6.20 1, cast located crucible former; 2, a plastic crucible former; 3, suspended crucible former.

around a metal crucible former or by cutting a circle of wax, removing a segment and joining the exposed ends (Fig. 6.20³).

2   The former is suspended over the centre of the cast with the point of the cone about 10 mm above the highest point of the pattern.

3   Primary sprue formers of 5·0 mm wax profile are curved in a posterior direction from the underside of the crucible former to the pattern. Secondary sprue formers are treated in the same manner (Fig. 6.20³).

Sprueing full plates

Full plates may be sprued using the suspended crucible method, with the sprue formers attached to the posterior border of the pattern. Alternatively, metal sprue formers (1·5–2·0 mm diameter) may be attached to the beading. Five are used, one in the centre of the anterior region with two along each side (see p. 90, Fig. 6.15). They are attached to the pattern by holding the wire (which should be about 3 cm long) in the fingers and warming one end over a Bunsen burner flame. (If it becomes too hot to hold, it is too hot to attach to the pattern.) The heated end is dipped into inlay wax then pressed into the beading (the thickest part of the pattern). It is held in position until the wax has set. Each sprue former is directed towards the centre of the pattern to join at a point about 2 cm above the highest point of the pattern. A hollow wax crucible former is placed over the sprue formers and sealed to them (see p. 90, Fig. 6.15). Reservoirs may be attached as required. It is essential that metal sprue formers are straight, because they have to be removed from the investment before heating can commence.

GAS VENTS

Vents are passages leading from the mould to the outer surface of the investment, for the purpose of expulsion of mould gases. They may be placed in the following areas:

1   Where two flows of metal are likely to combine (Fig. 6.20[1]).
2   At the extremity of thin areas (Fig. 6.20[1]).
3   At the end of clasps.

Care is taken with their placement otherwise metal will be lost through the vent.

Round profile wax (0·8 mm thickness) is generally used. One end is attached to the pattern, the other to the top edge of the crucible former or outer surface of an investment cast (Fig. 6.20). Molten metal acts like water to find its own level. Therefore its flow down a vent will stop when it reaches the level of the excess metal (the button) contained in the crucible.

7 Investing, Casting and Finishing Procedures

INVESTING PROCEDURES

When the pattern has been sprued and attached to a crucible former it is ready to be covered with investment material, the procedure being termed investing. A plastic or metal cylinder is used to support the investment material around the pattern.

Casting cylinders and their preparation

There are two main types of casting cylinder—a sealed metal cylinder, which is left around the investment material during the casting procedure, and a split metal or plastic cylinder which is removed once the investment has set. A sealed metal cylinder is used to support plaster bonded investment materials because the investment has a low impact strength. A split casting cylinder is used to support the ammonium diacid phosphate bonded investment materials which have a higher impact strength. The split design has a securing clip to prevent the cylinder opening during use.

Investment materials expand during the setting and heating procedure and therefore compensate for the contraction of molten metal as it solidifies. Allowance must be made for this expansion, when a sealed cylinder is used, by lining the inside of the cylinder. Asbestos liners were used in the past, but have more recently been replaced by paper liners. Unfortunately, paper liners burn away during the heating procedure, which necessitates careful handling if the investment block is to be prevented from falling out of the cylinder during the casting procedure.

1   A casting cylinder is selected with an internal diameter of at least 5–10 mm greater than the widest measurement of the pattern and about 10 mm higher.

2   The inside of a metal cylinder is lined with a piece of thick blotting paper or waxed crinkled paper. Its length is adjusted to the internal circumference of the cylinder and its height to about 5 mm less than the length of the cylinder. The liner edge should be level at one end of the cylinder and short at the other. A blotting paper liner is moistened to cause it to swell and also help it to adhere to the surface of the cylinder (see p. 90, Fig. 6.15). This also prevents the liner absorbing water from the investment. Waxed crinkled paper liners are waxed to the internal wall of the cylinder or held in position by paper clips.

3   Plastic cylinders are not lined but the securing clip is positioned and the internal join sealed with petroleum jelly, wax, or paper, to prevent investment clogging the inside of the clip, which would make removal difficult. Plastic cylinders are used in conjunction with plastic crucible formers.

Crucible formers

Crucible formers are produced in two basic outlines—a steep-sided cone, to be used when metal is to be cast into the mould by centrifugal force, and a shallow cone for use when steam or air pressure is to force the metal into the mould.

Cast located former

The crucible will have been formed in the cast during the duplication process. It is now necessary to fill the crucible with wax and raise the cast to allow new investment material to completely surround it and to prevent the investment filling the crucible. The crucible former is sealed to the base of the cast and to a 10 cm² base-board (it may be metal or hardboard). The crucible former should raise the base of the cast 5 mm off the board. Alternatively, the investment cast is placed on and sealed to a plastic crucible former which raises the cast to allow investment to surround it. The casting cylinder is positioned around the investment cast, with the pattern centrally placed, and sealed to the board. The cylinder edge, at which the liner is short by 5 mm, is placed in the region of the crucible former. This allows investment material to grip the cylinder and any resultant distortion will not affect the mould.

Suspended former

The crucible is suspended over the pattern by being fixed to the sprue formers as described in the previous chapter. Three wax cubes, about 5 mm² on each face, are waxed in triangular formation to the base of the investment cast and to a base-board. These allow complete coverage of the cast with investment material. The cylinder is placed around the cast, and sealed to the base-board. The end of the cylinder at which the liner is short, is placed in the region of the crucible former.

INVESTING PROCEDURE

Single stage method

The mixing of investment materials should follow the manufacturer's instructions. A small alteration in the powder–liquid ratio will result in a change in the expansion. About 400 g of powder is sufficient for an 8 cm (3 inch) diameter casting cylinder.

1   The investment is mixed to the manufacturer's recommended proportions, spatulated to a creamy consistency and vibrated to reduce air inclusions.

2   The cylinder is held in one hand with the fingers under the base and the thumb on the top edge of the cylinder. The back of the hand is placed on the electric vibrator whilst investment material is slowly poured down the inside wall of the cylinder. The cylinder is rotated from side to side at frequent intervals to dislodge air from around the investment cast and pattern.

3   When the cylinder is full, vibration is stopped and the cylinder placed on a shelf away from the vibrator.

Two stage method—with a cast

This method is used when a vibrator is not available or when an initial fine investment layer is required to form the surface of the mould. A second layer, consisting of a coarse permeable investment material, is used to complete the procedure. The casting cylinder is not placed around the pattern initially.

1 About 50 g of investment is mixed according to the manufacturer's instructions.

2 A fine paintbrush (about a No. 4) is wetted, and is then used to pick up an increment of investment and to paint it on to the surface of the pattern. Care is taken to prevent air being trapped. The procedure is repeated until the whole pattern has been covered with approximately 5 mm thickness of investment material. It is also extended beyond the pattern on to the cast and along the whole length of the sprue formers.

3 When the investment material has set, the cylinder is positioned and sealed to the base-board. A thin mix of coarse embedding investment is made. The thin consistency is required to facilitate wetting of the previous layer of investment and to ensure the casting cylinder is filled quickly and easily. A layer of liquid may develop on the exposed top surface of the investment which may be absorbed by sprinkling dry investment powder on to it. The investment is allowed to set.

Two stage method—without a cast

It is possible to adapt a wax pattern to a master cast, withdraw it and invest without the use of a duplicate investment cast.

1 Having formed the pattern, attached sprue formers (of which some should be metal to support the pattern) and crucible former, the pattern is removed from the cast whilst the area immediately adjacent to the pattern is lubricated lightly with petroleum jelly. The pattern is returned to the cast.

2 A mix of investment, about 50 g is generally sufficient, is spatulated and painted on to the pattern as described previously. This is allowed to set (Fig. 7.1).

3 The pattern is removed from the cast and the crucible former sealed to the base-board. A further 50 g mix of investment is made and painted on to the fitting surface of the pattern, covering the

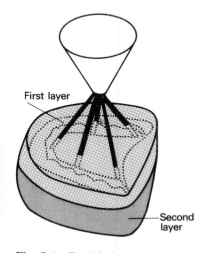

First layer

Second layer

Fig. 7.1 Double investment technique.

outer edges of the first layer of investment material. This is allowed to set (Fig. 7.1).

4   A lined casting cylinder is sealed around the pattern and filled with embedding investment material.

5   An alternative method is to remove the pattern from the master cast before covering with investment and to seal the crucible former to a base-board. It is surrounded by a lined casting cylinder which is then filled with investment material. This method requires considerable care and skill if distortion of the pattern is to be avoided.

Vacuum investing

The methods so far described are acceptable for plaster bonded investments but phosphate bonded investment materials are thicker and tend to set quicker, which makes it more difficult to eliminate air from them during the investing procedure. Elimination of air is achieved by covering the pattern with investment whilst under vacuum. There are various vacuum investing machines, all of which basically consist of a vacuum pump, mechanical spatulator with special mixing vessels and a vibrator. They may be bench-mounted or wall-mounted. A pipeline connects the vacuum pump to the top of the mechanical spatulator, the spindle of which interlocks into the drive spindle of the pump. The lid of the mechanical spatulator is an airtight fit on to the mixing vessel and contains a housing into which the casting cylinder is placed.

The investment powder and liquid are accurately measured according to the manufacturer's instructions and placed in the mixing vessel. The mechanical spatulator with the vacuum pipe attached, is positioned on the mixing vessel and the spindle of the spatulator interlocked with the spindle of the vacuum pump. The unit is switched on and air removed from the mix whilst it is spatulated. After about 20 seconds, the investment mix is vibrated whilst vacuum is continued. After 10 seconds of vibration, the casting cylinder is slowly inverted to allow the investment to trickle down its inside wall. Vibration is continued throughout and care is taken to prevent investment material being sucked into the vacuum pipe. Inversion is continued until the casting cylinder is sitting on the vibrator with the mixing vessel above it, at which point the cylinder will be full. The vacuum pump is switched off, the cylinder removed to a safe place and the various parts of the vacuum investor cleaned. Vacuum investing does not eliminate air inclusion completely, but does reduce it considerably.

CASTING PROCEDURE

Mould preparation

The crucible former is removed once the investment material has set. Metal crucible formers are firstly warmed (plastic ones are not heated), carefully twisted to break the seal with the investment and then pulled away from the cylinder. Loose particles of investment are brushed off.

The exposed end of each metal sprue former is heated over a Bunsen burner flame, the cylinder held with the sprue former facing downwards, the exposed end of the former is held in a pair of snipe-nosed pliers and rotated to loosen it. Once loose, the sprue former is pulled out of the mould, any loosened investment falling away from the sprue hole and not down it. A careful check is made to ensure the absence of dislodged particles of investment, since such particles could block the sprue hole and prevent entry of metal.

Split casting cylinders (metal and plastic) are removed at this point.

Heating the mould

The next stage is to heat the investment mould in a gas or electric furnace to:

1   Remove the pattern to form a hollow mould. This is accomplished in the following manner.

    a   The wax is softened.
    b   The wax ignites and burns.

c The wax leaves an impermeable carbon deposit on the surface of the mould.

d Further heating removes the carbon to produce a permeable mould surface.

2 Expand the mould which helps to compensate for the contraction of metal as it cools in the mould. Other forms of mould expansion take place:

a Setting expansion. This occurs as the investment material sets

b Hygroscopic expansion. This is an extension of the setting expansion which may be induced by the addition of water to the setting investment material.

The mould is positioned at an angle against the inside wall of the furnace with the sprue holes downwards. The temperature is raised to 700°C when plaster bonded investments are used and to 960–1040°C when phosphate bonded investments are used. All moulds should remain at this temperature for some time to allow it to 'heat soak'. This removes carbon from the surface of the mould, and ensures temperature and expansion uniformity throughout the mould. The length of the heat soaking time is adjusted in accordance with the manufacturer's instructions which may vary from 15 minutes to 60 minutes depending upon the size of the casting cylinder used.

Casting metal into the mould

There are various methods available for filling the investment mould with molten metal. Two methods only will be described.

Steam pressure

Steam pressure is produced by placing a damp pad over the crucible of a hot casting cylinder. The steam produced forces the molten metal into the mould. A machine which uses this method is the

Solbrig (Fig. 7.2). It is supplied with various sizes of base plate to suit different casting cylinders, and two sizes of pad container for the casting arm.

1   The pad container is removed from the casting arm and lined to a depth of 5 mm with a suitable water-absorbent material. Thick blotting paper, although not ideal will suffice. This must be discarded after use. A new liner is soaked with water. After a while, excess water on the surface of the pad is removed until moderate thumb pressure just causes moisture to ooze around the thumb. The container is returned to the casting arm.

2   For this technique, a metal casting cylinder must be used and left around the investment material. The preheated casting cylinder is removed from the furnace by use of metal tongs and placed on the casting machine. The casting alloy is placed in the shallow cone-shaped crucible above the sprue holes and heated with a blow-torch flame. As the temperature rises, the metal flows to the base of the

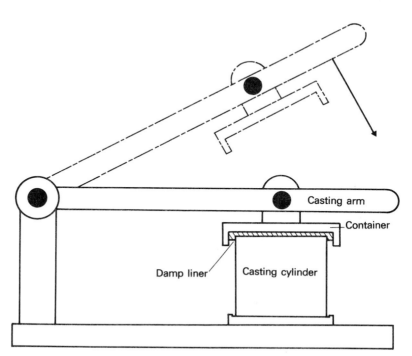

Fig. 7.2   Steam pressure casting machine.

crucible to cover the sprue holes. A powdered flux is sprinkled over the surface of the metal. Its function is to remove oxides from the surface of the metal and to prevent further oxidation. Flux is not added until the metal has covered the sprue holes, otherwise it may block them. Further heating of the metal eventually causes it to appear to spin. Heating is continued for a few seconds longer, to ensure complete fluidity, and then the casting arm is rotated downwards to press the moist pad on to the rim of the casting cylinder. The pad must not touch the molten metal because it will cool the metal before it has time to fill the mould. The pad is held firmly in position for about 30 seconds.

3 Upon raising the casting arm, excess metal, termed the button, will be seen in the crucible. The cylinder is put in a safe place until the button ceases to be red in colour, which takes about 5 minutes.

Centrifugal force

The variety of casting machines which use centrifugal force is quite large, but they may be categorized into two types: spring operated and electrically operated. The casting procedure is similar in both, therefore only the spring operated method will be described here. A horizontally rotating centrifugal casting machine consists of two arms which pivot at a central spindle. One arm contains a cradle for holding the casting cylinder and a separate refractory crucible in which the metal is melted, whilst the other arm carries a movable weight for balancing purposes (Fig. 7.3).

1 The cold casting cylinder and refractory crucible containing the required amount of metal, are placed on the casting arm. The weight is adjusted on the opposite arm to balance the machine to ensure even spin.

2 The best casting results are obtained by the mould trailing the direction of spin (see p. 92, Fig. 6.18): a groove is scribed into the surface of the investment to indicate the desired position of the mould in the casting machine. The investment mould and crucible are heated in the manner described.

3 Meanwhile, the casting machine is prepared, the spring is wound, the balancing arm is moved until slight pressure can be felt,

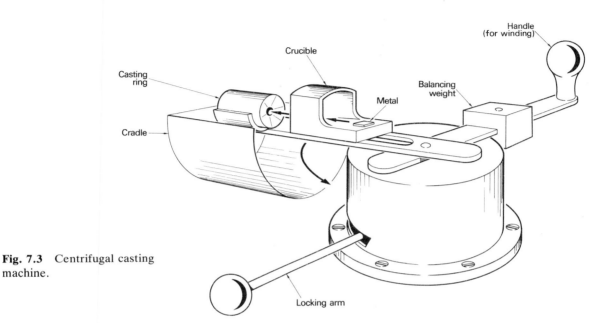

Fig. 7.3 Centrifugal casting machine.

and then given a maximum of five turns (this depends upon the size of the mould to be filled, large moulds require a greater number of turns) and the arms locked in position.

4 The heating apparatus to be used to melt the metal is prepared for use (see p. 106).

5 After the desired heating period, the crucible is removed from the furnace and positioned in the casting machine with the open end facing the operator. The metal is adjusted towards the top of the inclined floor of the crucible and a little flux sprinkled over its surface. The investment mould is placed in the cradle of the casting machine with the sprue holes facing the crucible. The position of the crucible is adjusted until it lies firmly against the mould.

6 Heating of the metal starts immediately. As the temperature rises, firstly the corners of the metal curl and then it slides down the inclined floor of the crucible. As heating progresses the ingots of metal combine, become spheroidal and appear to spin. A little flux may be added to the surface of the metal if it oxidizes. When the metal is completely molten, the heat source is removed, and simultaneously, the casting arm of the machine is released to thrust the molten metal into the mould.

7 When the machine stops spinning, the mould is placed in a safe place until the button loses its red colour.

Melting the alloy

The type of heating apparatus used depends largely upon the melting range of the alloy being melted. The available apparatus includes gas with compressed air or oxygen; hydrogen–oxygen generators; electric arc; and induction coil. Oxyacetylene may be used for melting cobalt–chromium alloys, but this is being superseded by electric arc and induction coil methods. Therefore, oxyacetylene will not be described.

Gas and compressed air

This is used almost exclusively for melting alloys with a melting range below 1000°C. The gases are passed along two separate tubes to a single jet nozzle, where they mix upon leaving the apparatus. Such apparatus is called a blow-torch and it contains taps for adjusting the flow of each gas.

1 Gas and air tube connections are checked. The gas control on the torch is turned to approximately quarter open, the control at the bench is fully opened and the gas ignited.

2 The air control is turned to fully open on the torch and adjustment made by turning the control at the bench. This prevents a build-up of pressure inside the pipe during the melting procedure, which could fracture the pipe.

3 The control taps are then adjusted to produce a flame with distinct gas zones, as shown in Fig. 7.4, the reducing zone is the hottest area and hence is used to melt the metal; it also prevents oxidation.

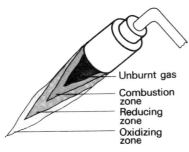

Unburnt gas
Combustion zone
Reducing zone
Oxidizing zone

Fig. 7.4 Zones of a blow-torch flame.

4 The casting machine is loaded in the manner described and the flame directed on the metal. The flame is slowly moved around the metal when large amounts are being melted to prevent overheating isolated areas. A dull appearance to the metal indicates incorrect use of the blow-torch flame has caused the metal to oxidize, whereas correct heating (using the reducing zone) produces a shiny appearance. The distance between torch and metal is adjusted until the surface of the metal takes on a shiny appearance.

5 An indication of fluidity is the apparent spinning of the metal. Heating is continued for a few seconds longer to ensure complete fluidity throughout the mass, and the casting machine is activated to thrust the metal into the mould. The control taps are closed on the torch and bench.

Gas and oxygen

This is similar in principle to the use of gas and air, but the higher temperatures obtainable make it possible to melt alloys with a melting range of up to 1200°C. The oxygen flow is controlled by a valve on the top of the oxygen bottle; the gas by a tap on the torch. Coloured protective goggles should be worn by the operator and onlookers.

1 After checking the security of the tube connections to the torch and oxygen bottle, the gas is turned on and ignited, and the oxygen pressure adjusted to 70–105 kN/m² (10–15 psi). The gas is adjusted to produce a light-blue flame about 2·5 cm long with a slight hissing sound coming from the torch.

2 The flame is directed on to the metal with the nozzle of the torch about 1·5 cm away from the metal. Complete fluidity should be obtained within 30 seconds, at which point the metal is thrust into the mould.

3 The oxygen is turned off and allowed to clear the pipeline before the gas is turned off.

Hydrogen and oxygen generator

This apparatus consists of an electrolytic cell which electrolyses water to produce hydrogen and oxygen. It is reported that the temperature of the flame can be adjusted by passing the gases through a liquid called a gas atomizer.

Table 7.1   Gas atomizers.

Gas atomizer	Obtainable temperature (°C)
Water	3300
Methyl ethyl ketone	1850
Acetone	1200

The gases pass along a single tube to a fine nozzle. Control is by switches on the generator casing.

1   The casting machine is loaded, the generator switched on and the gas ignited after about 5 seconds. Even with the largest nozzle supplied, the flame is no wider than a pencil lead and so it must be moved over the metal to obtain uniform heating. Small amounts of metal melt very quickly but the lack of width to the flame makes it difficult to heat large amounts of metal evenly.

2   When the casting procedure has been completed the control tap at the torch is turned off, and immediately after the generator is switched off.

Electric arc melting apparatus

This is used to melt the higher fusing alloys. The apparatus requires a high electrical input (30 A) which is used to create an electric arc at the end of two electrodes. The manufacturer's instructions should be closely followed because the arc can damage eyes and skin. The apparatus should be used in a separate room with facilities to prevent access of unprotected personnel during its use.

1   A current is selected according to which alloy is being melted, as indicated by the manufacturer's instructions. One electrode is attached to the negative terminal on the control box, the other to the positive terminal. The length of each electrode is set to approximately 10 cm and they are positioned about 5 cm apart.

2 The manufacturer's safety rules are rigidly followed. These generally include the use of a black apron to prevent glare, wearing of a specially designed facial visor, and the use of a foot switch in the electrical circuit which controls the current to the electrodes.

3 The operator puts on the apron and visor, then loads the casting machine.

4 The protective visor is pulled over the face which places the operator in complete darkness. The spring loaded electrode control is squeezed to bring the electrodes in contact and the foot control depressed. A brilliant arc is produced around the end of the electrodes which are adjusted until 3–4 mm apart.

5 The arc is directed on to the alloy which necessitates the ends of the electrodes being about 12 mm away from the alloy. High fusing alloys do not exhibit the same fluid characteristics as the lower fusing alloys. High fusing ingots should become rounded and show signs of collapsing, at which point they are thrust into the mould. The electrodes must be raised from the crucible before a centrifugal casting machine is set in motion.

6 The arc will be broken upon releasing pressure on the spring loaded electrode control and release of the foot switch. The protective visor is removed followed by the apron and the apparatus switched off.

Induction melting apparatus

This apparatus is included with an electronically operated centrifugal casting machine. Melting of an alloy is carried out by passing a high density alternating current through a coil of copper tube (Fig. 7.5). The polarity of the current alters from positive to negative at a rate of 1500 kHz. This produces a magnetic field around the coil. If an alloy, with the capability to have its polarity changed, is placed inside the coil, the rapid change of polarity produced causes the molecules of the alloy to oscillate and their molecular bonds to break down. This high intensity of molecular activity produces heat. The effect is that the alloy becomes molten and, in consequence, very hot. A cylindrical crucible is used and the process is ideal for cobalt–chromium alloys.

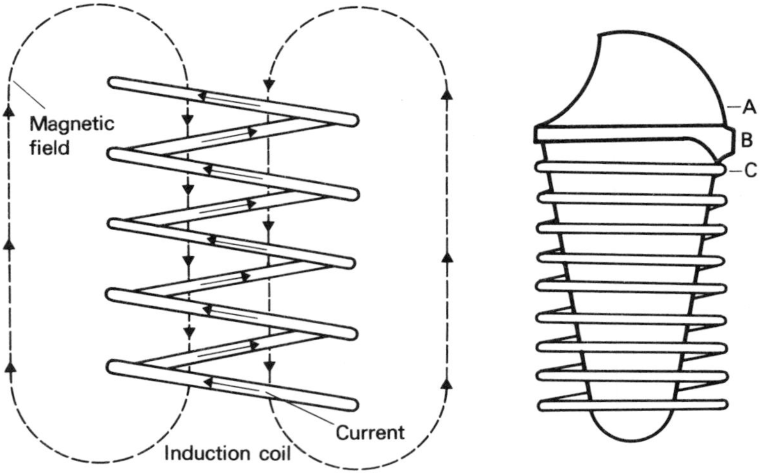

Fig. 7.5 Induction melting apparatus. A, crucible in which metal is melted; B, exit hole for molten metal; C, induction coil.

1   Water is circulated into the machine under pressure 138 kN/m² (20 psi). This travels through the copper coil to keep it cool during the melting process

2   The centrifugal casting arm is positioned over the copper coil and the coil raised to the undersurface of the casting arm. A localizing pin on the casting arm is used to ensure correct alignment and the coil is locked in position.

3   A circular crucible (Fig. 7.5) is seated in the machine and loaded with metal. Melting of the metal is viewed through a coloured visor. The starter switch is activated until the metal becomes red in colour, at which point the machine is switched off. The casting cylinder is loaded into the machine, and the starter switch reactivated. In about 30 seconds the metal will begin to sag and a circular shadow appears to hover over the metal. Eventually, the shadow will diminish in size towards the centre of the crucible and then disappear.

4   As the shadow disappears the induction coil is lowered and the casting machine activated to thrust the metal into the mould.

5   The electricity supply to the machine is switched off and the water supply turned off.

     A carbon crucible must be used when melting gold alloys. The crucible becomes hot and the heat is transferred to the metal to melt it.

Cleaning the casting

The mould should be allowed to cool on the bench for about 5 minutes in the case of a gold alloy button and for about 30 minutes when the alloy is of the cobalt–chromium type. The mould is quenched by total immersion in a bath of cold water. This causes plaster bonded investment to disintegrate which facilitates the removal of the casting. A knife is used on the inside of the cylinder, keeping it away from the casting, until the mould is free of the cylinder. The investment is prised off the casting, care being taken not to damage the casting and the remainder brushed off under running water.

Phosphate bonded investments are harder to remove from a casting, as they do not disintegrate upon quenching. The base and side of the mould are tapped by a mallet, which cracks the investment and causes it to fall away from the investment cast. It is now possible to tap on the head of the cast metal button to make the investment fall away from the casting. Small areas of investment adhering to the casting are removed by blasting with an abrasive medium.

Most castings exhibit an oxidized surface, and this is removed from gold alloys by acid, whilst cobalt–chromium alloys are cleaned by use of an abrasive medium.

Pickling solution

The removal of oxides from gold castings is termed pickling and a 50% dilute solution of hydrochloric or sulphuric acid is used. Normal safety precautions should be taken with acids.

1 The casting is placed in a heat resistant evaporating dish, covered with acid solution and heated over a Bunsen burner flame until the surface of the casting becomes clean. The acid should not be allowed to boil.

2   The casting is removed from the acid by use of a pair of plastic tweezers and rinsed under cold running water (metal tweezers should not be used because they contaminate the acid solution).
3   Oxide layers may also be removed by the use of sulphuric or nitric acid.

Ultrasonic cleaners

A more recent and safer method for removing oxides is the use of an ultrasonic cleaner. The casting is placed in a detergent solution in an ultrasonic bath and the solution subjected to ultrasonic vibrations. The vibratory waves act upon the surface of the casting to form bubbles which remove the oxides and investment. Cleaning is generally complete within 10 minutes, when it is removed from the solution and washed under cold running water.

Abrasive blasting

Traces of phosphate bonded investment and oxides on the surface of cobalt–chromium castings are best removed by blasting with an abrasive medium such as corundum. The blasting apparatus may be in various forms but essentially they consist of an air line containing a quick release valve and terminating in a nozzle. These are contained within a cabinet, the base of which is filled with abrasive medium; the front of the unit is inset with a viewing window and the side has an access hole with a flexible cover. The effectiveness of the blaster depends upon: the type of medium used (the medium, its particle size, surface irregularities, and hardness); the size of the nozzle through which the medium is blasted; air pressure used; and the distance between the object being blasted and the nozzle.
1   A protective rubber glove is worn on the hand holding the casting.
2   The apparatus is switched on. This automatically illuminates the interior of the cabinet of the apparatus and operates a dust extractor. The compressed air is turned on at a pressure of 400–550 kN/m² (60–80 psi).
3   The casting is inserted into the cabinet of the apparatus through

the access hole and the distance between the casting and nozzle adjusted to about 8 cm (never closer).

4   The valve is depressed by the free hand to release the medium under pressure. As one area is cleaned, the casting is moved to allow another area to be cleaned. The process takes about 3 minutes to clean the average casting when the blasting medium is new.

Casting failures

Failure to obtain a perfect casting is generally caused by a deviation from the correct technique. The most common failures are listed below.

Surface nodules

These may be found anywhere on the casting. They may be due to excessive use of a wax finishing agent which was still wet when the investing procedure commenced, and the trapping of air during the investing procedure. (Air bubbles—voids—fill with metal to become nodules on the surface of the casting.)

Small ridges

These are caused by movement of the casting cylinder during setting of the investment which results in cracks. They may be found on any surface of the casting.

Fins or fine feathery ridges

These are found anywhere on the casting and are caused by too rapid heating of the investment mould, which vaporizes the water in the investment which cracks the surface of the mould.

Rough surface to the casting

There are many reasons why the surface of a casting may be rough.
1   The pattern may have been dirty prior to investing.

2   Use of a coarse investment.

3   Overheating the mould causes the binder of plaster bonded investments to decompose in the presence of carbon at temperatures in excess of 700°C. The resultant disintegration causes roughness.

4   High casting pressures, caused by overwinding a centrifugal casting machine, may damage the mould surface.

Foreign body inclusions

Inclusions of investment or superfluous flux, are found in areas furthest from the point of attachment of sprues.

Distorted castings

A finished casting may be distorted due to any or all the following reasons:

1   The pattern may be distorted when withdrawn from a master cast, during the direct method of investing.

2   The mould may become distorted as the investment material expands, if a liner is omitted from the casting cylinder.

3   The mould may be undersize if not heated sufficiently to obtain the expansion required to compensate for the contraction of the metal.

4   The casting may be distorted during the cleaning and finishing procedures.

5   A duplicate investment cast may have been inaccurately produced.

Porosity

This is the reduction in density of a casting by the presence of voids due to the absorption of mould gases or the lack of precautions to compensate for alloy contraction

1   Localized or contraction porosity is found in the region of sprue attachment and is the result of thin sprues or sprueing to thin areas.

2   Subsurface porosity is caused by high mould temperatures or overheated alloy. It becomes apparent as the surface is polished during the finishing stage.

3   Back pressure porosity is found at the extremities of the casting where gases are slow to vacate the mould. A pressure is built up which prevents the metal filling the mould.

Incomplete castings

This may result from a faulty pattern, incorrect sprueing, gases in the mould causing back pressure, insufficiently heated mould, or incompletely melted metal. Also, during prolonged melting of an alloy, the mould can cool sufficiently to cause the metal to solidify before completely filling the mould.

FINISHING PROCEDURES

When a casting has been cleaned of investment and oxides, it is ready for the finishing procedure. It is advisable for all operators to wear protective goggles and to use dust extractors throughout these procedures. A face-mask should be worn when dust extractors are not available.

1   Removal of sprues. High speed electrical motors, capable of spindle speeds of at least 18 000 rev/min and preferably with an integral dust extractor, should be used. A 4 cm carborundum disc is attached to a Huey 304 mandril which in turn is locked into the chuck of the grinder. The grinder is rotated and the casting so positioned that the disc cuts into the furthest edge of the sprue away from the operator (Fig. 7.6). As the metal becomes hot it is quenched and the cutting procedure continued. Each sprue is removed in turn, as close as possible to the casting. Recontouring of the sprue area may be accomplished using the carborundum disc.

2   Irregularities on the fitting surface of gold castings are removed using a rose-head bur or a small cone-shaped stone. When phosphate bonded investments have been used the whole of the fitting surface is dressed by gentle grinding using a small cone-shaped

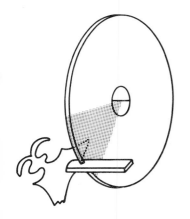

Fig. 7.6 The casting is so positioned that the disc cuts into the furthest edge of a sprue away from the operator.

stone. For cobalt–chromium alloys, this procedure is best accomplished by using an air turbine motor capable of 80 000 rev/min. Care must be taken not to overtrim, otherwise a poorly fitting denture base will result.

3 The denture base is shaped using stones. There should be no sharp edges to the casting and the surface to be polished should be smooth.

4 When satisfied with the shape and smoothness, the casting is placed on the master cast. The retentive area of a clasp arm will score the cast as it moves over the bulbous portion of the tooth; no other scoring should occur, if it does, the denture base must be modified.

5 Interdigitation with the opposing cast is checked for possible areas of interference and modified where necessary.

6 The fitting surface of a gold alloy casting is brightened by use of a rotating 2 cm (1 inch) wire brush. This is generally held in a handpiece and gradually moved over the surface of the metal. The fitting surface of the denture is then polished lightly with pumice in the manner to be described later.

7 The fitting surface of cobalt–chromium castings is electronically polished.

a The denture is thoroughly washed under cold running water, and then dried. The fitting surface is blasted with an abrasive and rewashed. From this stage onwards it is important that the fitting surface is unhandled because grease from the hand will prevent the electrolytic action.

b A wire electrode is securely attached to the casting and to the positive electrical terminal from the polishing unit control box.

c A negative terminal is attached to a non-reactive plate which is usually stainless steel. The negative plate is termed the cathode and the denture which is positive is termed the anode. The anode and cathode are placed no closer than 1 cm apart in an acidic solution called an electrolyte (see Appendix).

d The current is switched on and the voltage adjusted to 10 with an amperage of 1·0 for every square millimeter of denture area being electrolytically polished. About 2·5 A is sufficient for the average denture. Polishing takes 10–15 minutes depending upon the temperature of the electrolyte.

The surface of the denture is ionized and goes into solution. The result is a smooth bright surface. If the current density is too low, an etched surface will result, whilst a high current density rapidly reduces the thickness of the denture base.

8 The polishing stage is best carried out by investing the fitting surface of the casting in a block of plaster of Paris. This block follows the periphery of the casting and leaves the area to be polished exposed. The block enables handling, as the metal becomes hot during the polishing procedure, and prevents warpage.

9 It is now possible to smooth the casting using a hard rubber polishing wheel. It is moved over the metal continually, using a rotary movement to prevent the formation of facets. All scratches must be removed at this stage.

10 Polishing is carried out on a dental lathe, which should include a dust extractor. A partly worn black polishing brush is attached to the lathe spindle and the machine set to high speed. The brush is then impregnated with an abrasive polishing compound (see Appendix) and the denture base pressed firmly against the brush. The position of the metal is altered continually to prevent faceting. Felt cones and metal-centred brushes (4 cm in diameter) may also be used until the metal exhibits a dull smooth surface. The brushes are exchanged for a cloth polishing mop, which is impregnated with jeweller's rouge when polishing a gold alloy, or chromium oxide when polishing cobalt–chromium. The polishing procedure is repeated until a high lustre is obtained. The denture base is removed from the plaster block and the peripheral surface polished. Great care must be taken when polishing near clasp arms, which are easily distorted.

11 All polishing compound is removed by washing in a hot detergent or in an ultrasonic cleaner.

12 Finally, all traces of blocking-out wax are removed from the master cast by firstly, soaking the cast in warm water for about 10 minutes, and then secondly, using boiling water to remove the wax (a dry cast may fracture if directly submitted to boiling water). The denture base is then fitted to the cast ready to be presented to the surgery.

HEAT TREATMENTS

The physical properties of some alloys may be altered by heating them to specific temperatures, the procedure being termed heat treatments. The physical properties of cobalt–chromium alloys are adequate without any treatment, but gold alloys respond well to heat treatment.

Annealing

Annealing is a procedure whereby an alloy is heated to allow its internal grain structure to reorientate and produce an homogenized state. An alloy is annealed after polishing and before it is hardened by heat treatment.

The casting is placed on a refractory tray and placed in a preheated furnace at 700°C. This temperature is maintained until the metal is cherry-red in colour which takes 3–4 minutes. It is quenched in a bowl of cold water. Oxides which form on the metal are removed by pickling.

Precipitation hardening

An annealed casting may be submitted to further heat treatment to improve its physical properties. Careful control of the temperature encourages a specific alteration in the internal grain structure called precipitation (see Appendix). This procedure may take place in a furnace or in a salt bath.

Furnace procedure

Most manufacturers make recommendations for heat-treating their alloy. In the absence of these recommendations a furnace is heated to 450°C and the casting placed on a refractory tray, and inserted into the furnace. The furnace is allowed to cool to 250°C over a period of 30 minutes, when the casting is quenched. The rate of cooling governs the physical properties; a very slow cooling time produces a brittle alloy devoid of ductility.

Salt bath procedure

Salts of potassium nitrate and sodium nitrate when mixed in equal parts and heated, become liquid at around 200°C. The temperature may be raised to 400°C and the dry denture placed in the solution which is allowed to cool to 250°C, at which temperature the denture is removed. Salt baths are said to produce better physical properties, prevent oxidation of the alloy, are inexpensive and may be used repeatedly. The solution will explode when water is introduced (similar to the effect produced when water is dropped into hot fat), therefore, castings must be dry when inserted into the salts.

8 Wrought Metal-work

The metal-work procedures described so far have been firstly fabricated in wax which was used to form a mould into which metal was poured. Metal structures may also be formed by shaping metal whilst cold. It is referred to as wrought metal-work. The metal is purchased in profile form similar to the waxes, i.e. sheet, wire, bar and mesh and are mainly of stainless steel, although gold alloys may also be used.

SUPPORT UNITS

It is important to adapt wire to the occlusal surface of a tooth in such a way that space between wire and tooth, where particles of food can stagnate, is avoided. This is achieved by adapting platinum foil to the tooth and flushing solder between the metal and foil. Embrasure hooks and occlusal rests may be formed in this manner but onlays are rarely formed in this way.

Occlusal rests

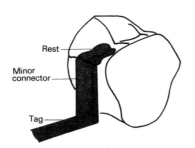

Fig. 8.1 Component parts of a wrought occlusal rest.

1   A D-shaped profile wire is selected and a piece placed on the occlusal surface of the tooth. A note is made of the high spots, which are ground away until the wire fits reasonably to the cast. The flat or curved surface of the wire may be placed against the tooth surface, depending upon the most appropriate contour.
2   The wire is bent at 90° to form a minor connector down the proximal surface of the tooth and a further right-angled bend to produce a tag (Fig. 8.1). The tag may be roughened in the manner of a lingual bar or closely adapted to other metallic components in readiness for soldering.

120

3   The occlusal rest is removed from the cast and a piece of platinum foil adapted to the occlusal surface of the tooth. It should be about 1 mm wider than the occlusal rest and be continued on to the proximal surface of the tooth for a distance of 1 mm. It must fit the cast accurately.

4   The occlusal rest is assembled on the foil and molten sticky wax flowed around it to form an integral unit with the foil.

5   The unit is removed from the cast, invested and soldered together (see p. 130). It is then ground to shape, smoothed and polished.

RETENTIVE UNITS

The principles of design for retentive units apply equally to wrought alloy clasps as they do to cast ones. Wrought metal clasps exhibit greater flexibility than cast metal ones, especially when round wire is used. This allows the use of a deeper undercut (0·75 mm is normal) and for a greater length of the retentive arm to be below the survey line.

1   The cast is surveyed in the normal manner, and unwanted undercuts eliminated. The cast is duplicated, and the duplicate surveyed to outline the bulbous portion of the tooth and to indicate the depth of undercut required. The position of the clasp is drawn on the tooth.

2   The type and cross-sectional shape of wire is selected. Gold alloy or stainless steel may be used in round or D-shaped cross-sectional form. The round wires are easier to adapt but their small area of contact with the tooth reduces their retention. D-shaped wires have improved retention because they cover more tooth area, but they are less flexible and more difficult to adapt.

3   Many types of pliers may be used for bending wrought metal clasps, but three popular types are (a) Adams Universal pliers, (b) loop-forming pliers and (c) Lowe–Young pliers (Fig. 8.2). The author prefers the Lowe–Young pliers; the ends of the beaks are similar to the loop-forming pliers but also contain grooves which are helpful when bending D-shaped wires through their cross-section.

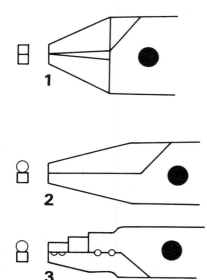

Fig. 8.2   1, Adams Universal pliers; 2, loop-forming pliers; 3, Lowe–Young pliers.

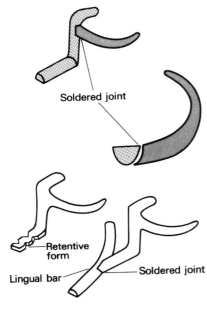

Soldered joint

Retentive
form

Lingual bar   Soldered joint

Fig. 8.3 A wrought clasp may be soldered to the minor connector of the occlusal rest. The tag may be roughened or soldered to another metal structure, such as a lingual bar.

4A   Bending round profile wire. A length of wire is cut and its end held in the beaks of a pair of pliers and bent around the round beak of the pliers. The angle of the curve will differ slightly from tooth to tooth. The wire is positioned against the tooth and the angle of the wire checked. It is bent to accurately fit the tooth. Bending commences at the tip of the wire, and the clasp positioned against the tooth after each bend to check its contour. (a) The clasp may be terminated on the proximal surface of the tooth and soldered to the minor connector of the occlusal rest (Fig. 8.3), (b) the proximal end of the clasp formed into a tag or (c) the clasp continued on to the lingual or palatal surface of the tooth to form the reciprocating arm. When the proximal end of the clasp is to be formed into a tag, the wire is closely adapted to the tooth up to the centre of the proximal surface and then bent at 90° to allow it to travel down the proximal surface of the tooth. Before this can be fitted against the cast, the wire must be given a further right-angled bend towards the saddle. The tagging should be at least 1 mm off the surface of the cast and so positioned as to be closely adapted to other metal-work when it is to be soldered to these metals. Alternatively, the end of the tag may be further bent at 90° towards the cast and excess metal cut off to leave a right-angled extension of 1 mm length.

4B   Bending D-shaped profile wire. These wires are firstly bent through their cross-section and then to the contour of the tooth with the flat surface of the wire against the tooth. It is important for the whole of the flat surface of the wire to contact the tooth, to prevent the formation of a stagnation area which could lead to the formation of caries.

5   Once adapted to the tooth, the end of the clasp is tapered. This shaping is minimal for round wire clasps but a D-shaped wire must be gradually tapered from about half-way along its length. The clasp is then smoothed and polished in the normal manner.

CONNECTORS

Lingual bar

The principles to be followed in constructing a wrought lingual bar

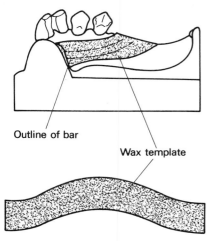

Outline of bar

Wax template

Fig. 8.4 A wax template is formed to assist with the contouring of a lingual bar.

are similar to those outlined for a cast lingual bar. A duplicate cast is advised in case the master cast is damaged during the subsequent stages.

Preliminary preparation

1 The position of the bar is outlined in pencil on the duplicate cast. Each end of the bar should enter a saddle area and terminate about three-quarters the way along the length of the saddle.

2 A piece of modelling wax is adapted to cover the outline of the bar drawn on the cast. Its lower edge is trimmed to finish on the lower outline of the bar (Fig. 8.4). The wax is removed to be flattened and become a template, delineating the cross-sectional contour of the bar (Fig. 8.4).

3 A further piece of modelling wax is softened, formed into a roll and adapted to the floor of the cast to form a platform on which to rest the bar. This is trimmed to the lower outline of the bar and then removed from the cast.

4 A piece of gauge 40 tin foil is adapted closely to the lingual aspect of the cast, and secured to it with wax. This prevents the cast being damaged during the adaption of the bar and relieves pressure from the tissues when the bar is fitted in the patient's mouth.

5 The wax platform is reseated on the cast and sealed to it.

Bar adaption

1 A suitable length of bar is cut and a pencil mark drawn at its centre. The bar is laid on the wax template to determine the degree of bend required. The bar is held in a pair of bar-bending pliers, the centre of the bar being aligned with the centre of the pliers which are slowly closed to bend the bar through its cross-section (Fig. 8.5). The curvature is checked with the template, and bending continued until the bar conforms to the wax template.

2 Alternatively, Levo bar-benders may be used. The bar is pushed through the hole in each of two benders, which are positioned about 1 cm apart. The benders are twisted in opposite directions to bend the bar (Fig. 8.6).

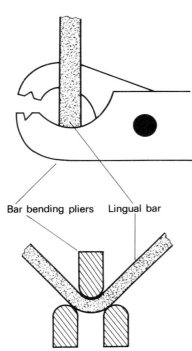

Fig. 8.5 Bar-bending pliers may be used to bend a lingual bar through its cross-section.

3 Levo bar-benders may be used to bend the bar to conform with the contour of the cast. Bending commences at the centre of the bar; care should be taken to ensure that the long axis of the bar lies in the same plane as the lingual contour of the cast, its shape and angle being checked by placing the bar on the wax platform.

4 The length of the bar is adjusted, the retentive form produced at the ends where they are to be encased in the saddles. Firstly, the ends are hammered flat, the bar being placed on an anvil and struck with a hammer. The shape of the bar must be checked on the cast, and the hammered area trimmed to prevent interference with the setting of denture teeth. Finally, grooves are cut to produce further retention, the angle of the grooves being such as to prevent the bar being pulled out of the saddle.

5 The bar is smoothed by use of a rubber wheel and polished in the manner described for cast metal-work. A plaster supporting block is not required during the polishing procedure. Polishing is postponed when clasps are to be soldered to a bar.

Sheet metal plate

The adapting of sheet metal to a cast is termed swaging. The methods available for swaging metal plates are:

1 Sheet metal is pressed on to a metal duplicate cast called a die.

2 Hydraulic pressure is used to adapt sheet metal on to a stone duplicate cast.

3 Explosive means are used to adapt sheet metal on to an araldite duplicate cast.

A popular method is the use of hydraulic pressure coupled with a stone die, and this method will be described.

Die preparation

The outline of the plate is drawn on the master cast, a post dam cut and the master cast duplicated in dental stone.

1 A length of triangular soft stainless steel wire is adapted to fit the post dam groove, with the longest edge of the triangle uppermost to

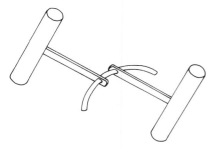

Fig. 8.6 Levo bar-benders may be used to bend a lingual bar.

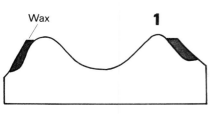

Wax **1**

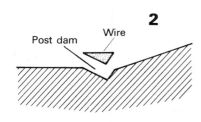

2
Post dam   Wire

Fig. 8.7 1, The buccal aspect of the cast is blocked out; 2, a piece of softened stainless steel wire is bent to fit the post dam.

come in contact with the plate (Fig. 8.7²). The wire is removed from the cast and put in a safe place until required.

2 The whole of the buccal and labial aspect of the cast is filled with wax from the sulcus to the outline of the plate on the alveolar ridge. It is helpful if a 1 mm ledge is formed at the edge of the outline of the plate (Fig. 8.7¹).

3 A spacer of one layer of modelling wax is formed to conform with the plate area.

4 A special tray is formed over the spacer in an autopolymerizing acrylic resin. As the tray is for use in the laboratory and not in the mouth, a short vertical handle only is required.

5 Upon completion of the tray, the spacer is discarded and the cast soaked in water for 10 minutes. The tray is filled with a thiokol rubber or silicone rubber impression material and an impression taken of the plate area of the cast.

6 A special die flask (Fig. 8.8) is prepared for use by lubricating its inner walls. The section without an internal lip is filled with plaster of Paris to within 5 mm of the rim and the impression tray inserted into it with the impression uppermost and its periphery level with the top of the rim of the flask. The plaster is smoothed, allowed to set and then lubricated.

7 A thick mix of die stone is made and carefully vibrated into the impression. The flask is assembled and filled with die stone through a hole in its base and the stone allowed to set.

8 The flask is opened, and traces of separating medium and loose particles of stone removed. A further die is poured in die stone.

Swaging procedure

Briefly the swaging apparatus consists of a cabinet containing a reservoir of oil, a large swaging flask with facilities for bolting its two sections together and a one-way valve for applying oil under pressure to the inside of the flask, and a pump for delivering the oil under pressure.

1 The duplicate cast and its surrounding stone within the flask is now referred to as the die. The second die to be poured is seated within its flask in the housing of the swaging flask (Fig. 8.9).

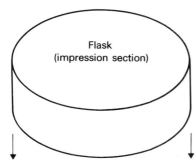

Flask
(impression section)

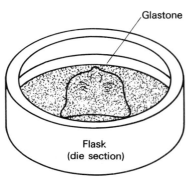

Glastone

Flask
(die section)

Fig. 8.8 A die is formed within a cylindrical flask.

2 Two holes, 5 mm deep, are drilled into the die about 5 mm buccal of each tuberosity. The post dam wire is checked for position on the die and its ends bent and cut to fit into the holes.

3 A disc of metal is selected. The metal is normally extra low carbon stainless steel plate in the form of discs 12·5 cm in diameter and 0·25, 0·50 or 0·75 mm thick. The thickness of metal selected depends upon the depth of the palate (Fig. 8.10). A metal plate is thinned by the action of swaging, the thinning being greatest with a deep-vaulted palate. Therefore, 0·25 mm thick plate is swaged on to a shallow palate, 0·5 mm thick plate on to an average depth of palate and a 0·75 mm thick plate is swaged on to a deep-vaulted palate.

4 The plate is centrally placed on the die. A sealing 'O' ring is positioned in the counter section of the swaging flask which in turn is located on the lower portion by use of a localizing pin. High tensile steel bolts are placed in each of twelve holes in the upper portion and screwed by hand into the lower section. Final tightening is accomplished by use of a torque wrench at 275 kN/m² (40 psi) and the bolts tightened in a diagonal sequence to produce even pressure.

5 A pipeline is attached from the pump to the one-way valve in the upper section of the flask and compressed air fed to the pump. The pump activator is depressed to force oil down the pipeline and on to the steel plate in the flask. The pump produces a pressure 100 times greater than the incoming pressure, therefore, 550 kN/m² (80 psi) input produces 55 000 kN/m² (8000 psi) output. The speed of the pump decreases as the pressure increases, until maximum pressure is attained, when the pump stops automatically. A high pressure swages quickly but can split a plate if the palate is deep. A low pressure only partially swages a plate to the cast. The plate is then removed from the flask, annealed to release stresses in the plate and returned to the flask for further swaging.

6 When the pump stops, it is deactivated and the pipeline released from the flask. The bolts are unscrewed and the flask opened. Oil present in the palate of the plate is drained off and the plate dried on a piece of cloth.

7 Excess metal is removed to 2 mm outside of the outline of the plate by use of a plate cutter. Final trimming is accomplished by use

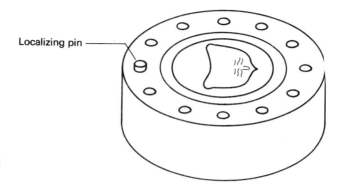

Localizing pin

Fig. 8.9 Die within the swaging flask.

of a carborundum wheel mounted on a lathe. The posterior border of the palate is trimmed at a later stage.

8 The soft stainless steel post dam wire is removed from the die, positioned to the undersurface of the plate and spot welded to the plate. Each weld must overlap the previous weld. The edge of the wire is ground to blend into the plate, the posterior border of which is trimmed to size and shaped.

9 A finishing bead is bent out of the triangular softened stainless steel wire and adapted to the plate, to which it is attached by overlap spot welding. The wire is ground to blend into the plate. When correctly welded and shaped, the post dam and finishing bead should be indistinguishable from the plate.

10 Tagging may be welded to the plate in the form of wire loops or mesh. Welding and shaping often result in slight warpage of the plate, therefore the plate is finished to the rubber wheel stage and then reswaged.

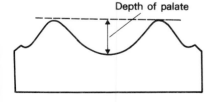

Depth of palate

Fig. 8.10 A disc of metal is selected according to the depth of the palate.

11 Before annealing is carried out, the plate is coated with a medium to prevent discolouration of the metal surface. The plate is thoroughly cleaned in an ultrasonic cleaner or washed by use of a degreasing agent such as Swarfega. It is essential that the metal is not touched by hand from this stage onwards. The plate is dried and coated with Berkatect. This is toluene-based, and therefore, dries quickly.

12 The plate is annealed. A furnace is preheated to 1050°C, the plate placed in the furnace for 3 minutes, and then immediately quenched in cold water. The Berkatect is self-descaling, and drops off the plate as a grey ash.

13 The plate is assembled on the die which was poured first and the palate filled with a small piece (1 × 2 cm) of 2 mm thick Neoprene. These are covered by a 9·0 cm (3½ inch) disc of 3 mm thick Neoprene which is further covered by a 12·7 cm (5 inch) disc of 1·5 mm thick Neoprene. The swaging flask is assembled and the swaging process repeated.

14 Finally, the plate is given a high polish by use of a universal polishing compound followed by chrome oxide. (Jeweller's rouge is not used on stainless steel because iron oxide—rouge—deposits left on the surface of the plate produce rust spots after the denture has been worn.)

SOLDERING PROCEDURE

The joining of two metals by use of a third metal possessing a lower melting range than the metals to be joined is termed soldering. Successful soldering is accomplished by following certain principles rigidly.

Principles of soldering

1 *The units to be joined must be clean of grease and oxides.*
The surfaces of the metal should be abraded by use of a rotating bur, or rubbed with sandpaper to remove oxides. Final cleaning may take place in a dilute acid solution (HCl for gold alloys and Aqua Regia for stainless steel) or by use of an ultrasonic cleaner.

2 *The units to be joined should be in close proximity.*
A very small space should exist between the metal units to be joined to allow the metals to expand without causing distortion when heated. The space should be equal to the thickness of a piece of tissue paper which produces the appearance of the units being in contact, but when held to a light source leaves a space just visible between the surfaces. This results in the physical forces of capillary attraction drawing the molten solder along the joint.

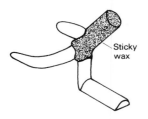

Fig. 8.11 The units are removed from the cast by holding the extending roll of sticky wax.

3 *The units should be firmly and accurately localized.*

A clasp arm adapted into a tooth undercut is difficult to remove from a cast without producing some distortion, especially when joined to other units, therefore, the retentive portion of the clasp arm is firstly freed from the undercut by bending the arm away from the tooth. Sticky wax is used to join the units and a short rod of sticky wax sealed to them (Fig. 8.11). The units are removed from the cast by holding the extending rod of sticky wax.

4 *The minimum of investment should be used.*

Large amounts of investment take a long time to heat. During a long heating procedure metal units can oxidize and this oxidation will impair the flow of solder. Investment should be approximately 5 mm larger than the area of the components involved.

5 *The joint should be completely accessible to the blow-torch flame.*

Solder always flows to the source of heat. Therefore, if only the top of a joint is accessible to a flame, the solder will not penetrate to the undersurface. Investment is cleared from the immediate vicinity of the joint either by trimming or by covering the undersurface of the joint with wax prior to investing.

6 *A flux is always used.*

Fluxes prevent the formation of oxides on metal. The joint should either be fluxed prior to localization or before the metals are heated. The use of flux is kept to a minimum. Borax is perhaps the most commonly used flux, for gold work and, although excellent in use, it does have the disadvantage of swelling when heated (efflorescence). This can dislodge units to be joined, resulting in distortion. A potassium fluoride flux is used on stainless steel.

An antiflux may be used to confine solder to the joint. This has the effect of making the metal dirty which prevents solder alloying with the components. Grease, graphite and an oxidized surface all act as antifluxes.

7 *Heating the investment block.*

The investment block should be heated to a dull red colour throughout, before solder is introduced to the joint. Solder will form into a sphere and oxidize if prematurely added, and will not flow.

8 *The minimum of solder is used.*

The strength of a soldered joint relies upon an alloying of the solder with the units being joined. This alloying takes place microscopically on the surface of each metal. Therefore, assuming the units being joined have been correctly shaped and are in close proximity, the minimum of solder will be required. Solder should be introduced to that area of the joint furthest from the source of heat, so that it will travel along the joint by capillary attraction towards the heat source.

9 *The heat source is removed immediately soldering is complete.* The flame is removed from the work immediately the joint has been satisfactorily filled. Overheating will cause the base metal constituents of the solder to vaporize and cause the solder to pit. Overheating also effects the physical properties of the metals being joined.

10 *The oxides and flux are removed.*
Those areas of an appliance which have not been fluxed or covered with investment material invariably oxidize during the heating procedure and these oxides must be removed. Equally, flux remaining in the region of the soldered joint must be removed. This is accomplished by pickling in acid or immersion in an ultrasonic cleaner.

Soldering procedure

1 The units are adapted to the cast and to each other, the space between them being adjusted to the thickness of a piece of tissue paper. The abutting surfaces and about a 1 mm area surrounding them are cleaned by grinding with a stone or rubber wheel. This is followed by pickling in acid or cleaning in an ultrasonic cleaner. The abutting areas should not be touched by hand from this stage onwards.

2 The units are reassembled on the cast and sticky wax flowed along the joint. A short rod of sticky wax is softened, and placed over and sealed to the units. This produces a solid joint and a rod which may be gripped to withdraw the components from the cast. The undersurface of the joint should be filled with wax to prevent investment penetrating it which would prevent solder filling the joint.

3 A coarse-grained embedding investment, specially manu-factured for the soldering procedure, may be used, or alternatively casting investments give satisfactory results. The investment material is mixed to a thick consistency, placed on a lightly lubri-cated surface and the appliance embedded into it. There should be about 5 mm of investment, at least, beneath the metal, otherwise the block may fracture during subsequent procedures. Clasps should be completely covered, with the exception of the joint, but there is no necessity to invest the whole of a plate or bar. (About 10 mm either side of the joint is sufficient area to cover with invest-ment.) The components should be covered with about 2·5 mm of investment. Thinner sections may fracture during heating pro-cedures and thicker sections conduct heat from the joint, prolong-ing the soldering procedure.

4 When the investment has set, the sticky wax is chipped off and traces of wax removed by pouring boiling water over the investment block. Investment is removed from around the joint to make it accessible to the flame (Fig. 8.12). Care should be taken not to remove too much investment in these areas, because it will weaken the joint.

5 The joint is fluxed at this stage. A small amount only is used. Careful application of the flux will confine the solder to the joint. Unfluxed areas readily oxidize, thereby acting as an antiflux to prevent solder flowing over areas where it is not required.

6 The investment block is heated by placing it over a Bunsen burner flame, in a furnace, or by use of a blow-torch flame. All metal components, such as plates and bars need to be embedded completely in investment if either of the first two methods are to be adapted, otherwise distortion may occur. The temperature of the furnace is raised slowly to 700°C. The blow-torch method is quicker, but does not produce an even rise in temperature. A brush flame is directed on to the work and moved around the investment block twice, then removed for about 10 seconds, and the procedure repeated. Eventually, steam will rise from the investment which can cause the block to fracture if heating is too rapid.

7 When the investment is dry, the blow-torch flame is directed continually on to the investment. Care is taken not to overheat thin

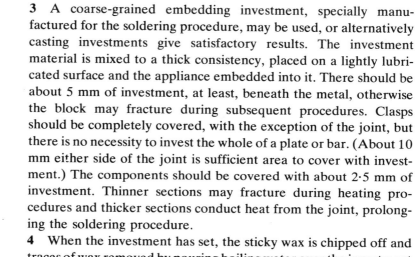
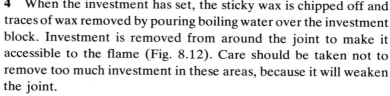
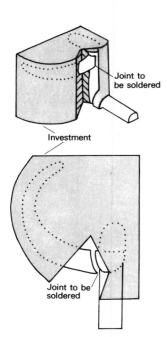

Fig. 8.12 Investment material is removed from around the joint to make it accessible to the flame.

components whilst waiting for thicker units to reach the required temperature. The flame must be kept moving over the whole investment block. When the block reaches a dull red colour, the flame is reduced to the diameter of a pencil (the gas and air pressures are reduced) and this flame directed on to the joint only. Solder is added to that side of the joint furthest from the flame. If the temperature is correct, the solder will flow immediately. Further solder is added until the joint has been filled, when the flame is withdrawn.

8   The soldered appliance is allowed to cool until it loses its heat colour and then quenched by total immersion in water. The investment is removed and the oxides and flux cleaned off the metal by pickling in acid or by use of an ultrasonic cleaner. The appliance is repolished.

An alternative method is the use of a hydrogen oxygen generator unit to solder the units whilst positioned on the cast. This eliminates the necessity to localize and invest. The units are secured to the cast by small increments of plaster of Paris placed over clasp arms etc, and only the joint area is heated. The flame is directed on to the thicker component until the metal is a dull red colour and then the thinner component brought up to the same temperature. Solder is introduced to the joint in the normal manner. Since there is no investment to heat, most operations can be completed in less than 1 minute.

Stainless steel is more difficult to solder than gold, carbides forming readily on the surface of the metal when it is heated. A special flux—potassium fluoride—must be used and this is added to the joint before the metal is heated. Once carbides form, they can be removed only by blasting with an abrasive medium or grinding; flux will prevent their formation but not remove them. Fortunately, stainless steel can be joined by an alternative method known as welding.

WELDING PROCEDURE

The procedure of welding stainless steel consists of passing an electric current through the steel which offers resistance to flow of the current. This causes the temperature of the metal to rise and the metal to become soft. Pressure is applied to the metal which causes the components to bond together. The current and pressure are applied by thin electrodes to one spot of the metal at a time, from which the technique derives the name spot welding and the machine is called a spot welder.

The pressure, current and duration of current are controlled on most spot welders and these are adjusted according to the thickness of metal being welded. The units are held in the operator's hands and positioned between the electrodes of the welder. When the foot control or hand control is depressed, an electric current is passed through the electrodes, which simultaneously exert pressure to the spot involved. The actual weld is said to be achieved in about 1/200th second with modern spot welders (see Appendix).

9 The Setting of Teeth

The process of positioning teeth on a base is termed setting up. Its purpose is to improve or restore masticatory efficiency, to restore speech and to restore or improve the patient's appearance. Whilst fulfilling these functions the teeth must not interfere with the oral musculature or affect the retention of the denture base during use. This has led to the establishment of basic positions for teeth based upon the average jaw relationship. Although students are advised to follow these positions, it should be understood that they are modified according to the patient's individual requirements.

INSTRUMENTS

The instruments required for the setting of teeth are: a wax knife, a Le Cron wax carver, an Ash No. 5 wax carver, or pen point trimmer, a pair of dividers and a 10 cm² ceramic tile. A toothbrush with shortened bristles is required to produce a stippled effect in the wax and a pledget of cotton wool for polishing the wax.

TOOTH SELECTION

The dental surgeon selects the mould, size and shade of teeth required for each patient. This is done at the chairside by study of the shape of the patient's face, the length and mobility of the upper lip, the vertical dimension and the distance between the canine eminences. When considering the partially dentate mouth, the available denture teeth are compared with the standing teeth. The shade of teeth is selected by comparison with the standing teeth or by facial complexion and age of the patient. Men generally have

134

darker teeth than women and the natural dentition tends to darken with age. Posterior teeth are generally the same shade as, or slightly darker than, the canines. They should be narrower buccolingually than the natural dentition and the anteroposterior width should be such that the last molar finishes on the anterior border of the retromolar pad or tuberosity. This subject is dealt with in detail in most clinical textbooks.

TRANSFERENCE OF INFORMATION

When teeth are set on an occlusal rim the information recorded on the rim is destroyed. Consequently it is desirable to transfer the information to the mounting plaster on the articulator.

1   The centre line is continued in a gingival direction and scribed into the mounting plaster (Fig. 9.1).

2   A pair of dividers is opened an arbitrary amount, the tip of one arm pressed into the mounting plaster along the scribed centre line

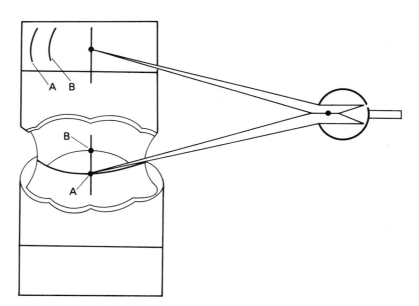

Fig. 9.1   Information recorded on the occlusal rim and base is transferred by the use of a pair of dividers to the mounting plaster.

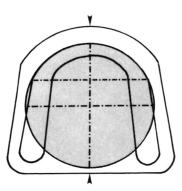

Fig. 9.2 A Bonwell circle.

and the tip of the other arm rested on the low or normal lip line. This measurement is scribed on the top or the front of the mounting plaster (Fig. 9.1).

3 The dividers are adjusted to record the high lip line in the same manner (Fig. 9.1).

4 The vertical dimension is established on an articulator by adjustment of a screw at the rear of a simple hinge articulator, and by the incisal guidance pin on an anatomical articulator.

5 It is possible to record the labial contour of the upper occlusal rim by use of a Bonwell circle. After selection of the teeth the dividers are set from the mesial edge of the central to the distal edge of the canine on the same side. The dividers are then used to cut a circle of wax (Fig. 9.2). In the majority of cases it will be found that the circle exhibits the same curvature as the anterior surface of the occlusal rim. Its use will be described later (see p. 139).

SETTING TEETH TO OCCLUSION

When learning to set teeth, it is helpful to consider jaws as having a static relationship only. A class I jaw relationship (Fig. 9.3) may be regarded as the ideal relationship with the teeth being set in the following manner.

Upper anterior teeth

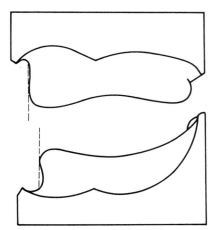

Fig. 9.3 A class I jaw relationship.

1 The upper cast is removed from the articulator and the upper occlusal rim separated from the lower.

2 The Bonwell circle is divided into four equal segments by scribing a cross through its centre and then a further line scribed about 6 mm from the centre (Fig. 9.2). The centre of the posterior border of the cast is marked with pencil lead, and the circle laid on the occlusal surface of the upper rim with the single line bisecting the cast from the centre line anteriorly to the mark scribed on the posterior border of the cast. It will be seen that the circle approximates with the labial surface of the rim and the most anterior line scribed on the wax is just posterior of the canine lines.

3   The basic positions of teeth may be described in relation to three criteria: 1, the occlusal or horizontal plane; 2, the vertical plane or axis; 3, the alveolar ridge.

3.1   Central incisor (Fig. 9.4).

> **a**   The incisal edge should lie parallel with and be on the occlusal plane.
>
> **b**   Its labial long axis should be 90° to the occlusal plane, hence parallel with the vertical plane and centre line.
>
> **c**   Its long axis, when viewed from the proximal surface (its proximal long axis) is about 8° from the vertical with the neck of the tooth nearer the alveolar ridge.
>
> **d**   The relationship of the tooth with the alveolar ridge is determined by the labial and occlusal surfaces of the occlusal rim.

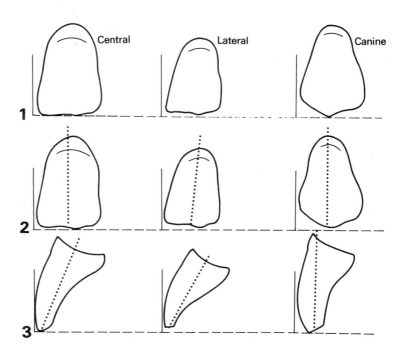

Fig. 9.4   Relative position of anterior teeth to: 1, the occlusal or horizontal plane; 2, the vertical plane; 3, the combined horizontal and vertical planes.

3.2   Lateral incisor (Fig. 9.4).

    a   The incisal edge should lie parallel to the occlusal plane but about 1 mm above.
    b   Its labial long axis should be about 10° from the vertical with the incisal edge nearest to the centre line.
    c   Its proximal long axis is about 12° from the vertical with its neck slightly nearer the alveolar ridge than the central incisor.
    d   Relationship with the alveolar ridge is determined by the occlusal rim.

3.3   Canine (Fig. 9.4).

    a   The centre of the incisal edge only (the cusp point) should contact the occlusal plane.
    b   Its labial long axis should be perpendicular or parallel with the centre line.
    c   Its proximal long axis is perpendicular, which produces a slight prominence of the neck of the tooth.
    d   The canine should lie over the canine eminences which are seen as slight prominences on the labial surface of the alveolar ridge of the upper cast.

4   The upper occlusal rim and base is assembled on the cast and the occlusal surface of the rim placed on a ceramic tile to check for an even contact with the tile.

5   The tile is removed, a wax knife heated over a Bunsen burner flame, and a section of the rim removed from the centre line to the canine line. It is firstly removed at an angle from the occlusopalatal edge of the rim to the high lip line, followed by a reduction in occlusal height of about 3 mm (Fig. 9.5).

6   The central, lateral and canine teeth relating to the carved area of the occlusal rim, are removed from the tooth card and cleaned of carding wax.

    The cast is held in one hand which is positioned with the index finger resting on the top of the bench peg. The blade of a wax knife is heated, the tip of the third finger of the hand holding the knife is rested on the occlusal surface of the rim and the wax softened by making cuts into the carved area. It may be necessary to reheat the

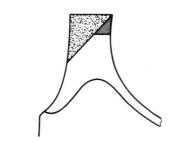

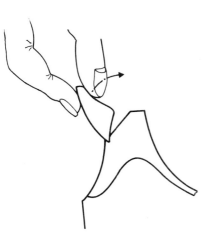

Fig. 9.5   The occlusal rim is trimmed in two stages, the wax softened and the tooth positioned.

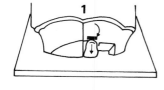

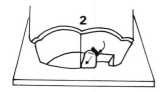

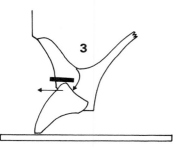

Fig. 9.6 Adjusting the position of a tooth to: 1, lower the incisal edge; 2, twist the tooth; 3, increase the prominence of the neck of a tooth.

knife several times before softening is completed. The knife is discarded and the central tooth gripped with the incisal edge between thumb and index finger (Fig. 9.5). The tooth is positioned neck first, the mesial edge resting along the centre line, then the incisal edge moved palatally to align with the occlusal rim. Excess softened wax will be displaced incisopalatally. The tooth position is checked by placing the occlusal rim on the tile. If the incisal edge is too long, slight pressure on the tile will compress the tooth into the wax. Other adjustments, outlined below, may be made, but the wax must be resoftened on the side of the tooth to which it is to be moved before the adjustments are carried out.

a *Incisal edge short of the occlusal plane*. The wax around the palatal aspect of the tooth is resoftened and the occlusal rim placed on the tile. The wax knife blade is inserted into the wax at the centre of the neck of the tooth and the blade twisted in a clockwise direction to force the tooth downwards (Fig. 9.6[1]).

b *Change of labial vertical axis*. When the wax knife blade is placed slightly mesial of the centre of the neck of a tooth and twisted anticlockwise, the neck will move away from the centre line and the distoincisal corner will drop.

If the blade is placed slightly distal of the centre of the neck of a tooth and moved in a clockwise direction, the neck will move towards the centre line and the mesioincisal tip will drop (Fig. 9.6[2]).

c *Neck too prominent*. The neck of a tooth may be depressed by firstly softening wax behind the tooth, then pressing the neck inwards.

d *Neck depressed*. The neck of a tooth may be made more prominent by placing the blade of a knife behind the tooth and twisting (Fig. 9.6[3]).

7 The position of a tooth in relation to the labial contour of the occlusal rim is checked by removing the tile and laying the Bonwell circle on the occlusal surface of the rim. The tooth should follow the contour of the circle (Fig. 9.7). Adjustment is made by holding the incisal edge of the tooth between finger and thumb and twisting. Its relation to the occlusal plane is checked by use of the tile.

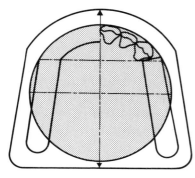

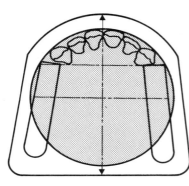

Fig. 9.7   The Bonwell circle is used to check the symmetry of the teeth being set.

8   The lateral incisor tooth is positioned in the same manner. Its mesial edge should contact the distal edge of the central, and the tile and Bonwell circle used to check its position.

9   The procedure is repeated for the canine. Its mesial edge contacts the distal edge of the lateral. All three teeth are sealed to the base by melting the wax around them.

10   The above procedure is repeated to set the other central, lateral and canine, which should simulate the positions of the teeth already set. The tile and circle are used throughout to ensure uniformity and conformity to the occlusal plane and the contour of the occlusal rim. The distal edge of the canines should be symmetrical when compared with the lines drawn on the Bonwell circle (Fig. 9.7).

11   The speed of operation may be increased by softening wax in the region of the central, lateral and canine teeth at the same time, positioning these teeth quickly by eye, and then checking and adjusting their positions against a tile and Bonwell circle. The technique is repeated on the opposite side of the cast.

Upper posterior teeth

The basic positions of the posterior teeth are described in relation to the three criteria mentioned for the anterior teeth.

1   First bicuspid (premolar) tooth (Fig. 9.8).

   a   The apex of the buccal cusp should contact the occlusal plane.
   b   The buccal long axis should be parallel to the vertical plane.
   c   The proximal long axis should also be parallel to the vertical plane.
   d   The palatal cusp should be 0·5 mm away from the occlusal plane.

2   Second bicuspid (premolar) tooth (Fig. 9.8).

   a   The apex of the buccal cusp should contact the occlusal plane.

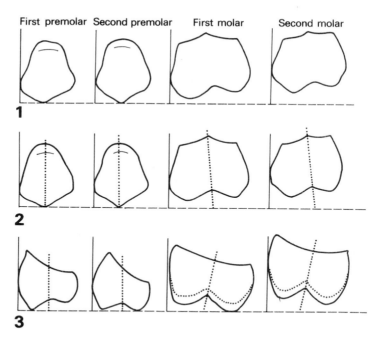

Fig. 9.8 Relationship of posterior teeth relative to:1, the occlusal or horizontal plane; 2, the vertical plane; 3, combination of the horizontal and vertical planes. The dotted cuspal outline on the molars indicates the position of the posterior cusps of each tooth.

b The buccal long axis should be parallel to the vertical plane.

c The proximal long axis should be parallel to the vertical plane.

d The centre of the palatal cusp should contact the occlusal plane.

3 First molar tooth (Fig. 9.8).

   a The apex of the mesiobuccal cusp should be about 0·5 mm from the occlusal plane.

   b The apex of the distobuccal cusp should be about 1·0 mm from the occlusal plane.

   c The buccal long axis will be approximately 5° from the vertical plane.

   d The centre of the mesiopalatal cusp should contact the occlusal plane.

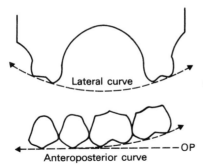

Fig. 9.9 The compensating curves.

e The centre of the distopalatal cusp should be approximately 0·5 mm from the occlusal plane.

f The proximal long axis will exhibit a deviation in a buccal direction of about 5° from the vertical plane.

4 Second molar tooth (Fig. 9.8).

a The centre of the mesiobuccal cusp should be approximately 1·5 mm from the occlusal plane.

b The centre of the distobuccal cusp should be approximately 2·0 mm from the occlusal plane.

c The buccal long axis exhibits a deviation of approximately 15° from the vertical plane.

d The centre of the mesiopalatal cusp should be approximately 1·0 mm from the occlusal plane.

e The distopalatal cusp should be about 1·5 mm from the occlusal plane.

f The buccal long axis exhibits about a 15° deviation from the vertical plane.

It should be evident now that the posterior teeth are set to two curves (Fig. 9.9); an anteroposterior curve and a buccopalatal or lateral curve (see Appendix). They are referred to as the compensating curves. They compensate for the downwards, forwards, and lateral movements which take place at the condyles. Failure to produce such curves would result in partial loss of contact between the teeth of opposing jaws during function, which could result in loss of retention of the denture bases.

1 The occlusal rim is trimmed by the dental surgeon at the chairside to record the muscular neutral zone and so the buccal wall of the rim indicates the line to be followed by the buccal cusps of the posterior teeth. The anteroposterior dimension of the premolars plus an extra 2 mm is marked on the occlusal rim immediately posterior to the canine, and wax removed to allow setting of the premolars. The height of the rim is reduced by about 4 mm, and the sides chamfered from the centre of the rim to a line level with the neck of the canine on both buccal and palatal surfaces. This produces a tapered rim, indicating the approximate centre of each tooth (Fig. 9.10).

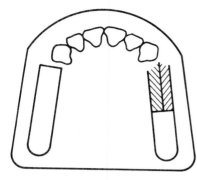

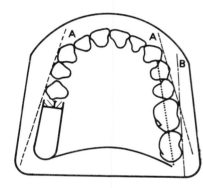

Fig. 9.10 The occlusal rim is tapered; A, the canine, premolars and edge of the occlusal rim should be in a straight line; B, the buccal surface of the molars should form a straight line.

2 Wax is softened in the first premolar region, and the tooth positioned neck first, followed by adjustment of the occlusal surface on the tile. It should contact the canine. A straight edge is placed against the bulbous labial surface of the canine, and the buccal wall of the occlusal rim and the premolar adjusted to contact it (Fig. 9.10).

3 Wax is softened in the area of the second premolar, the tooth being set as described above and contacting the adjacent premolar. Its buccal wall should contact the straight edge resting against the canine and occlusal rim (Fig. 9.10).

4 The molar region of the occlusal rim is trimmed in the manner described for the premolars. Wax is softened in the first molar region and the tooth positioned with its mesial proximal surface contacting the second premolar. The mesiobuccal cusp of the molar should contact a straight edge projected along the buccal walls of the premolars.

The distobuccal cusp is displaced slightly palatally from the straight edge. This should result in the occlusal sulci of the premolars and molars being in a straight line (Fig. 9.10). The tooth is aligned to the vertical and horizontal planes.

5 After softening of the final area of wax, the second molar tooth is set with the buccal wall tapering towards the palate (the degree of taper depends upon the shape of the teeth used) (Fig. 9.10). The important criterion is that the occlusal sulcus should be in line with that of the other posterior teeth (Fig. 9.10). The tooth position is adjusted to the vertical and horizontal planes.

The procedure is repeated on the opposite side of the occlusal rim. It should be remembered that the posterior teeth have been set to the compensating curves, which results in the molar teeth being away from the horizontal plane. Care should therefore be taken to ensure that the anterior teeth and premolars contact the horizontal plane during the setting of the last molars.

Lower posterior teeth

Setting of the lower teeth commences with the first molar tooth, which governs the position of the remaining teeth in relation to the upper posterior teeth. The upper cast and wax denture are assembled on the articulator. The lower occlusal rim is removed from the cast and a line drawn along the centre of the posterior ridge. The line is extended from the posterior to the anterior region of the cast (Fig. 9.11). The retromolar pad is normally lingual of this line and the sulci of the posterior teeth are set along the line.

1 The lower occlusal rim is sealed on to the cast and the articulator closed. A mark is made on the lower rim corresponding to the centre of the upper canine. A second mark is made, corresponding to the distal aspect of the upper first molar. The height of the rim is reduced between the marks and the edges tapered, the peak of which lies directly over the ridge (Fig. 9.11).

2 The wax is softened in the molar region and the first molar positioned so that the centre of the tooth lies directly over the ridge, with the occlusal surface approximately level with the occlusal surface of the rim. The articulator is closed to bring the tooth in contact with the upper molar. The mesiobuccal cusp of the lower molar should be anterior to the upper molar and contacting the distal aspect of the second premolar. This results in the mesial development groove being directly beneath the mesiobuccal cusp of the upper molar and the distal development groove beneath the distobuccal cusp of the upper molar (Fig. 9.12). The buccal cusps of the upper molar should overlap the buccal cusps of the lower molar. There should be contact between upper and lower teeth on both the buccal and lingual aspects.

3 The articulator is opened and wax softened in the second premolar region. The tooth is positioned centrally over the ridge, its occlusal surface level with that of the molar and its distoproximal surface contacting the molar. The articulator is closed and the premolar adjusted to contact the upper premolar teeth.

4 Wax is softened in the first premolar region and the tooth positioned. It should contact the proximal surface of the second lower premolar and cusp with the mesial aspect of the upper first premolar.

5 The procedure is repeated on the opposing side of the cast.

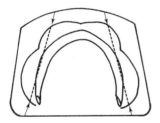

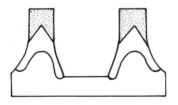

Fig. 9.11 A line is drawn along the alveolar ridge and the occlusal rim trimmed to a point which should lie directly over the line.

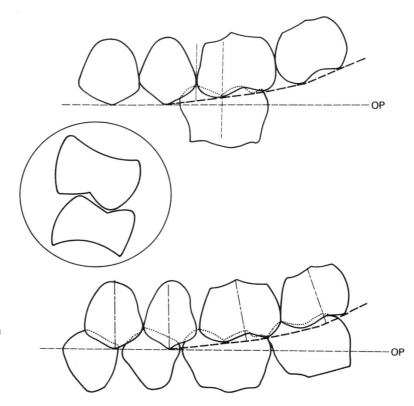

Fig. 9.12 The mesial development groove of the lower molar lies directly beneath the mesiobuccal cusp of the upper molar. The buccal long axis of each tooth should be at 90° to the compensating curve. The insert shows the mesiodistal view.

6 Finally, the occlusal rim is trimmed and softened in the second molar regions and each tooth positioned.

It will be found that the buccal long axis of each tooth is at 90° to the compensating curve (Fig. 9.12).

Lower anterior teeth

The lower anterior teeth are last to be positioned. The labial aspect of the occlusal rim indicates the position of the labial surface of these teeth and the degree of horizontal overlap (overjet) required. (This is the distance between the palatal aspect of the upper anterior

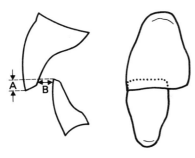

Fig. 9.13 A, vertical overlap; B, horizontal overlap.

teeth and the labial surface of the lower anterior teeth, Fig. 9.13.) The labial aspect of the occlusal rim is normally anterior of the lower alveolar ridge and follows the curvature of the upper anterior teeth. A slight modification in the position of the lower anterior teeth from the contour of the occlusal rim is permissible, according the amount of vertical overlap (overbite) necessary. The vertical overlap is the amount by which the upper anterior teeth overlap the lower anterior teeth (Fig. 9.13). The vertical overlap is generally in the region of 1–2 mm. A large horizontal overlap requires a large vertical overlap. This is discussed more fully under balanced articulation (see p. 148). The approximate relationship of the lower anterior teeth with the vertical and horizontal planes and the alveolar ridge are:

1 Central incisors (Fig. 9.14).

   a The incisal edge should be 1–2 mm above the horizontal (occlusal) plane to produce a vertical overlap.
   b The labial long axis of the tooth should be parallel to the vertical plane.
   c The proximal long axis of the tooth may exhibit a 5° labial inclination.

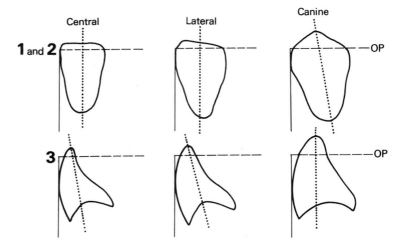

Fig. 9.14 The relationship of lower anterior teeth relative to: 1, vertical plane; 2, horizontal plane; 3, a combination of vertical and horizontal planes.

d The alveolar relationship is determined by the lower occlusal rim, but for stability of the denture base, the long axis of the incisors should be directed through the centre of the alveolar ridge.

2 Lateral incisor (Fig. 9.14).

a The incisal edge of the lateral normally corresponds to that of the central incisors.
b The labial long axis should be parallel to the vertical plane.
c Although the proximal long axis of this tooth exhibits a labial inclination it is normally less than that of the central incisors.

3 Canine teeth (Fig. 9.14).

a The incisal edge should be about 1 mm higher than that of the central and lateral incisors.
b The labial long axis should lean slightly to the midline of the denture.
c The proximal long axis should exhibit a slight lingual inclination or be completely vertical.

The procedure adopted to set the teeth in the wax occlusal rim is as follows:

1 The occlusal rim is trimmed to receive the anterior teeth. The height of the rim is reduced by about 4 mm, and the labial surface is chamfered to a point level with the necks of the premolars.

2 The wax is softened in the area of one canine and this tooth positioned in the manner described for the upper anteriors. Its cusp should be aligned with the interstitial area between the upper canine and lateral (Fig. 9.15). The position of the canine is important, failure to observe its relationship with the upper teeth generally leads to difficulties when setting the incisor teeth.

3 The wax on the opposing half of the rim is softened and the second canine positioned.

4 Each lateral incisor tooth is set in turn.

5 Finally the central incisor teeth are positioned.

The position of the teeth is adjusted to follow the curvature of

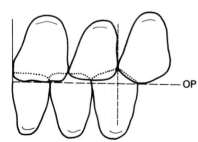

OP

Fig. 9.15 The cusp of the lower canine should be aligned with the interstitial area between the upper lateral and canine. OP, occlusal plane.

the upper anteriors with a vertical overlap of about 1 mm and a horizontal overlap of about 1–2 mm. When the procedure of setting teeth is complete the wax is smoothed and contoured in the manner described on p. 158.

BALANCED ARTICULATION

The procedure so far described, deals only with the ideal positions of teeth to ensure occlusion. As mentioned, occlusion is a static relationship but the oral cavity is dynamic and the dynamic relationship between teeth is called articulation. It may be defined as the intimate contact of as many opposing teeth as possible during masticatory movements. That part of the dentition involved in mastication is called the working side, whilst other contacting teeth are referred to as the balancing side (Fig. 9.16).

Table 9.1   Balanced articulation.

Masticatory (working) side	*Reciprocal (balancing) side*
Left	Right
Right	Left
Anterior	Posterior

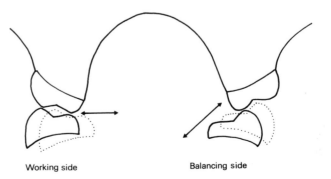

Fig. 9.16   That part of the denture involved in mastication is called the working side, whilst other contacting areas are called the balancing side.

Working side   Balancing side

Balanced articulation offers many advantages over occlusion: it produces improved occlusal contact, which distributes occlusal forces over a wide area of the oral tissues; there is reduced trauma to the oral tissues; denture stability is improved; masticatory efficiency is improved; and chairside time required to fit dentures is often reduced. Balanced articulation is best achieved on an adjustable condylar path articulator but some balance can be achieved on an average value articulator.

Principles of balanced articulation

Balanced articulation depends upon the following inter-relationship:

The condylar guidance (condylar angle)

This is the path of movement followed by the condyle on the balancing side as it moves downwards and forwards. The condyle on the working side moves slightly outwards and backwards (the Bennet shift) but many articulators do not allow for this movement and so rotation is about a fixed axis on this side. The angle of movement is different for every patient, and is a fixed factor for that patient. All other factors must be adjusted to the condylar angle.

The occlusal plane

This is a fixed factor once it has been determined by the dentist.

Incisal guidance

This is the glide which takes place in the anterior region during the downwards and forwards movement of the mandible required to bring the lower incisor teeth into gliding contact with the upper incisor teeth (Fig. 9.17). The angle may be calculated mathematically.

1 Calculate the average horizontal condylar angle, $(29° + 31°)/2$.

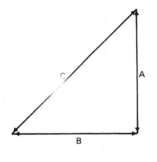

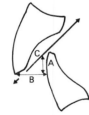

Fig. 9.17 The incisal guidance may be considered as the hypotenuse of a right-angled triangle. A, the vertical overlap; B, the horizontal overlap; C, the incisive guidance.

(Both angles would be the same for an average value condylar angle articulator.)

2 Double the cuspal angle, (20° × 2).

3 Subtract the smaller figure from the larger,

$$(20° \times 2) - \frac{(29° + 31°)}{2} = 10° \text{ incisive angle.}$$

This angle is taken as an arbitrary measurement for initially setting the incisal table on an articulator. The angle is adjusted during the positioning of the lower anterior teeth to harmonize with the rotating arc of the articulator (see p. 151) which allows the anterior teeth to have gliding contact. It is adjusted by increasing the vertical overlap which affects the appearance of the finished dentures.

Cuspal angle

Cusps can be considered as having two angles, the buccopalatal or lateral angle, and the anteriorposterior angle.

Balanced articulation is dependent upon the cuspal angles being parallel to the path of movement of the mandible, or, in laboratory terms, being parallel to the rotating curve of the articulator. This necessitates an increase in the steepness of the cusps from the premolars backwards to the last molar. Their angles must be increased with an increase in the condylar guidance.

1 The lateral cusp angles of the buccal cusps of the upper posterior teeth and the lingual cusps of the lower posterior teeth on the working side, should harmonize with the rotating movement at the condyle. This results in their inclination being flat when compared with the inclination on the balancing side (Fig. 9.20).

2 The lateral cusp angles on the balancing side must harmonize with the downwards and forwards movement of the condyle. This results in the palatal cusps of the upper posterior teeth and the buccal cusps of the lower posterior teeth, being parallel to the arc of rotation. These cusps have a steep inclination when compared with those on the working side (Fig. 9.20).

3 The anteroposterior cusp angle must harmonize with the downwards and forwards movement of both condyles as the mandible

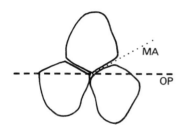

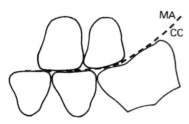

Fig. 9.18 The cuspal angle may be reduced by introducing a compensating curve. OP, occlusal plane; CC, compensating curve; MA, movement arc.

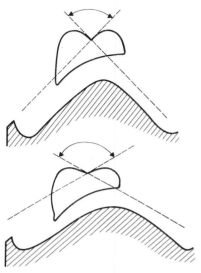

Fig. 9.19 The cuspal angle of teeth is modified according to the angle of the ridge.

moves into a protrusive position. These angles must be increased from the premolars to the last molar as the condylar guidance increases (Fig. 9.18).

4   A restraining factor which limits the steepness of the cusps is the retention of the denture. The resultant lateral forces associated with steep cusps produce high displacing forces at the fitting surface of the denture. These must be resisted by the walls of the alveolar ridge. A high alveolar ridge can resist high lateral displacing forces; as the ridge height decreases, so its resistance to lateral displacing forces decreases. Therefore, in the interest of stability, the cusp angle is reduced according to the ridge height (Fig. 9.19). This introduces a problem in that it has been said earlier that a steep condylar guidance requires steep cusps, and if the cusp angle is reduced in the interests of stability, cuspal contact will be lost during function making balanced articulation unobtainable. This problem can be overcome by the introduction of compensating curves.

Once teeth with a given cusp angle have been selected, balance is a matter of adjusting the posterior teeth to align the cusp angles to the rotation arc of the articulator, which results in the teeth being set to a curve—the compensating curve.

Compensating curve

Positioning of teeth is simplified by selecting an arbitrary compensating curve and adjusting it to align the cusp angles to the rotating arc of the articulator. Technically, reference is made to the adjustment of the compensating curve, when in reality the adjustment is being made to the cusp angle to align it to the rotating arc of the articulator and, hopefully, to the path of movement of the articulator. In terms of the compensating curve it can be stated that:

1   The compensating curve is increased with an increase in the condylar angle.
2   The compensating curve is increased with a decrease in cuspal angle.

Setting teeth to balanced articulation

1 The upper posterior teeth are set to an arbitrary compensating curve described earlier (see p. 140) and the lower first molars positioned. The buccal cusp of the lower molar should be parallel to and be in contact with, the palatal cusp of the upper molar. The lower lingual cusp should be parallel to the buccal cusp of the upper (Fig. 9.20).

2 The lower arm of the articulator is moved to left and right to verify contact between the opposing cusps.

3 If contact is lost, correction is carried out by:

  a Loss of cuspal contact on the balancing side.

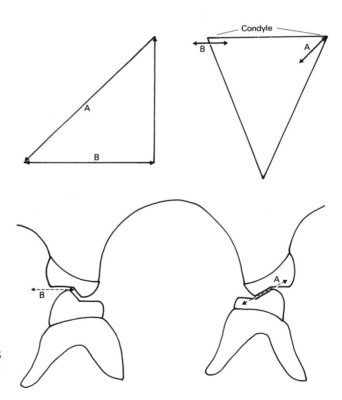

Fig. 9.20 Cuspal angles should lie parallel to the path followed by the mandible. A, direction of movement on the balancing side; B, direction of movement on the working side.

Action. Move the upper arm of the articulator laterally and adjust the buccal cusps of the lower molar tooth to contact the palatal cusps of the upper molar tooth. Open the articulator whilst still in the lateral position and seal the lower tooth to the lower base. Allow the wax to harden. Still with the articulator open, soften the wax, securing the upper posterior tooth on the side where the lower tooth has been adjusted. Close the articulator in centric relation. The upper tooth will be adjusted by the pressure from the lower tooth. Check for balanced articulation in left and right excursion.

b Contact between the palatal cusps of the upper molar tooth and the buccal cusps of the lower molar tooth, when representing the balancing side, but loss of contact upon becoming the working side.

Action. Lower the buccal cusps of the upper molar tooth until contact is achieved. This may also require the buccal cusps of the lower molar being lowered.

4 It is essential that the incisal guidance pin remains in contact with the incisal guidance table during movements of the articulator. Loss of contact indicates imbalance and the above adjustments must be made.

5 There should be cuspal contact when the articulator simulates protrusive movement. Failure to maintain cuspal contact in the posterior region requires an increase in the anteroposterior compensating curve in the following manner:

a The distal cusps of the upper molars are raised without altering the tooth's lateral inclination.

b The lower molar is adjusted accordingly. Care is taken to avoid alteration to the lateral compensating curve.

6 The premolars are set after the first molar has been set to balanced articulation.

7 The lower anteriors are set to the established balance. The vertical overlap being adjusted to allow the incisal edges of the lower teeth to glide over and just contact the incisal edges of the upper teeth when subjected to a protrusive movement.

If repeated attempts to obtain balanced articulation by modification of the compensating curve prove ineffective, high spots on cusps may be removed by spot grinding. This is carried out on:

a   The buccal cusps only of the upper posterior teeth.
b   The lingual cusps only of the lower posterior teeth.
c   The lingual aspect only of the upper anterior teeth.
d   The labial surface only of the lower anterior teeth.

As a memory aid this sequence is referred to as the BULL rule.
B: *B*uccal cusps of the
U: *U*pper teeth and the
L: *L*ingual cusps of the
L: *L*ower teeth.

INFERIOR RETRUSION

So far, setting up has been concerned with an ideal jaw relationship where intercuspation of teeth is comparatively easy. Unfortunately, this situation seldom exists in practice. Jaw relationships can vary from a gross inferior retrusion to a gross inferior protrusion. The term inferior refers to the lowest of two anatomical structures, in this case the one furthest from the skull. Therefore, an inferior retrusion is a receding mandible. When the mandible is a normal size but the maxilla is larger than normal, the relationship becomes a superior protrusion. Both jaw relationships come into the class II category (Fig. 9.21) which is distinguishable by (a) the lower ridge being well posterior of the upper ridge, and (b) the posterior region of the lower alveolar ridge may occasionally cross the upper ridge, to assume a buccal position. This is referred to as a cross-bite and is encountered to varying degrees. A cross-bite is not necessarily accompanied by a class II anterior jaw relationship.

The following procedure is used to set the teeth to a class II jaw relationship.

1   After mounting the casts on an articulator, the jaw relationship is analysed to determine the degree of the class II relationship.

2   Lower posterior teeth are selected which have a narrow buc-

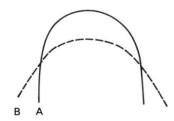

Fig. 9.21   Class II jaw relationship; A, upper alveolar ridge; B, lower alveolar ridge.

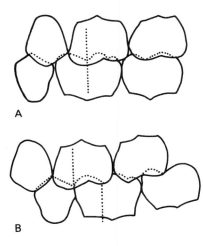

A

B

Fig. 9.22 Posterior tooth relationship in: A, class I and, B, class II jaw relationships.

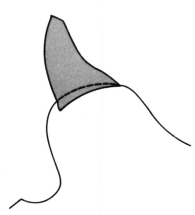

Fig. 9.23 The cast is trimmed to a depth of 1 mm in the labial area and tapering towards the crest of the ridge.

colingual dimension. These prevent the patient biting the tongue or cheeks.

3 The upper anterior teeth are set within the muscular neutral zone. This may entail fitting them to the labial surface of the alveolar ridge (see gum fitting, below).

4 It is permissible to exchange the first upper premolars for canines, in extreme cases. This is because the palatal cusp of the upper first premolar interferes with the lower canine when the mandible moves laterally.

5 In extreme cases, the first molar may be one unit posterior of the class I position (Fig. 9.22).

6 It is permissible to leave the lower first premolar off the denture to enable the rest of the teeth to be set over the alveolar ridge.

7 It is usual to increase the vertical overlap in an attempt to improve the patient's appearance and means of incising food. Incisal contact is often impossible when the patient's horizontal overlap is large. Therefore, the lower incisors are raised to allow food to be incised against the palatal surfaces of the upper incisor teeth or against the upper palate.

8 A lower incisor tooth may be left off the denture when space is restrictive.

Gum fitting

This term refers to the procedure of setting anterior teeth to fit accurately to the labial surface of the alveolar ridge and omitting a labial flange. It is required when a flange would distort the patient's facial contours.

1 The dental surgeon trims the occlusal rim to indicate the position of the labial surface of the anterior teeth and removes the labial flange to indicate that the teeth are to be gum fitted.

2 The lingual aspect of the neck of the central incisor is ground to fit the cast.

3 The tooth is positioned on the occlusal rim with its labial surface slightly prominent of the rim. A mark is scribed on the cast around the neck of the tooth by use of a sharp instrument. The tooth is removed and the cast trimmed to a depth of 1 mm within the scribed area, tapering away towards the crest of the ridge (Fig. 9.23). After softening the wax, the tooth is repositioned with its labial surface in the required position.

4 The procedure is repeated for each anterior tooth. Posterior teeth are set in the normal manner.

Retention is greatly impaired by this method of setting teeth but it may be improved by the use of labial extensions (wings) placed in the sulcus area (Fig. 9.24).

INFERIOR PROTRUSION

This is when the mandible is prominent. A normal mandible accompanied by a recedent maxilla is a superior retrusion. These come within the class III category of jaw relationships. It is distinguishable by (a) the incisor region of the lower is anterior to the upper alveolar ridge, and (b) the posterior region of the lower alveolar ridge is buccal to the upper ridge (Fig. 9.25).

Although the general principles of setting teeth are followed, a few modifications may be required.

1 After mounting the casts on an articulator, the occlusal rims and bases are removed and the jaw relationship studied.

2 Flat cusped or inverted cusped posterior teeth with a narrow occlusal table are selected.

3 The incisal guidance table is adjusted to 0°.

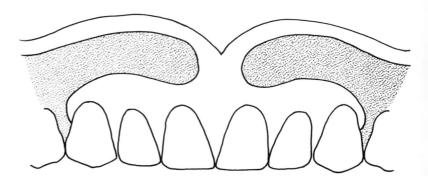

Fig. 9.24 Labial extensions (wings) aid retention.

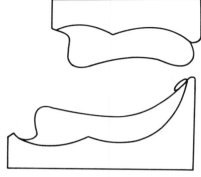

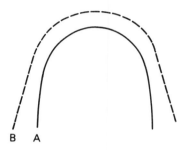

4 The upper anterior teeth are set in the normal manner.

5 The upper posterior teeth are set to a steep compensating curve; the lateral curvature being steeper than the anteroposterior curvature.

6 The lower first molar is positioned a full unit anterior to the class I position (Fig. 9.26) in extreme cases. The intercuspation of the mesiobuccal cusp of the lower first molar being mesial to the second upper premolar. Alternatively, the lower first molar may occupy its class I position and an extra lower premolar tooth set on each side of the denture.

7 Although the long axis of the lower anterior teeth should pass through the long axis of the alveolar ridge, it may be necessary to produce a slight lingual tilt to reduce the mandibular horizontal overlap in extreme cases.

8 The space available for the lower anterior teeth is large in these cases and so larger anterior teeth may be used, within reason, or an extra incisor tooth or a slight diastema may be incorporated.

9 A large cross-bite introduces difficulties when attempting balanced articulation, because the buccal cusps of the lower posterior teeth are outside the cusps of the upper posterior teeth. This difficulty may be overcome by the use of special cross-bite teeth which have a modified angle between the buccal and occlusal surfaces.

Fig. 9.25 Class III jaw relationship; A, upper alveolar ridge; B, lower alveolar ridge.

SETTING TEETH TO ABRASIVE RIMS

It is difficult to obtain balanced articulation when the articulator lacks the facility for lateral movement. A degree of balance can be obtained by setting teeth to the surface of an abrasive occlusal rim. The method outlined below is used with flat cusped teeth only.

1 Wax upper and lower occlusal rims and bases are used to mount the casts on an articulator, and the upper anterior teeth set to the prescription given by the upper rim.

2 The lower abrasive rim is placed on the lower cast and the upper posterior teeth set in such a manner that the cusps contact the occlusal surface of the lower rim.

3 The lower teeth are set to the upper teeth.

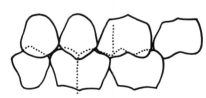

Fig. 9.26 Posterior tooth relationship in a class III jaw relationship.

SETTING TEETH ON A PARTIALLY DENTATE BASE

The setting of teeth to a partially dentate mouth follows the principles described for full dentures. The shape, size and mould of the natural dentition is reproduced. Although posterior teeth should be smaller than the natural dentition, their reduction should not allow the cheeks or tongue to collapse into the muscular neutral zone where they could become trapped by the dentition.

The position of anterior teeth is determined by the natural teeth, rather than by the occlusal rim. When their position conflicts with the principles of setting up, a compromise is sought in an attempt to achieve balanced articulation. It is sometimes impossible to obtain balanced articulation because of cuspal locking. In these instances balanced articulation may be achieved only after clinical modification of the occlusal table, by inlays or onlays cemented to teeth or by the attachment of onlays to the dentures.

THE WAXING PROCEDURE

When teeth have been set, the wax surrounding them is rough and irregular. This is smoothed and given the characteristic contour of the tissue surrounding the natural dentition. The procedure of adding and contouring wax is called waxing up.

Gingival contour

The gingival contour of the natural dentition should be carefully studied. It may be observed that:
1   The gingival contour rises and falls at intervals and does not present an even appearance (Fig. 9.27).
2   The gingiva is a roll of smooth tissue.
3   The gingiva is slightly concave between teeth where it becomes fastened to the alveolar bone.

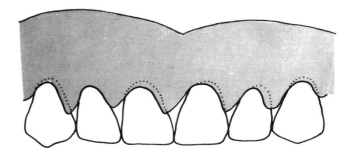

Fig. 9.27 The gingival contour rises and falls at intervals.

4   The gingiva may recede to expose the root of a tooth and the interdental papilla may become rounded with an increase in the patient's age.

Restoration of facial contour

The labial surface of the upper base is used to restore the patient's facial contour. This is generally accomplished by thickening the base around the neck of the canines and also slightly around the neck of the central incisor teeth. Such contouring should take the form of the roots, but since it is unusual for the root of laterals to be visible in the mouth, they are omitted from the denture base. This forms a slight depression over the laterals, known as the lateral fossa. The labial tissue of the natural dentition is not smooth but has a stippled appearance somewhat like orange peel. Stippling exhibits the following characteristics:

1   It is sparse over prominent root areas.
2   It is most prominent where the tissue is loose between the roots of teeth.
3   It diminishes towards the gingival tissue.
4   It is sparse towards the sulcus.

Retentive form

Periphery. The denture base is closely adapted to the periphery of a cast which has been poured from a muscle-trimmed impression. The denture base is trimmed free of muscle attachments if the cast has been poured to a non-functional impression.

Polished surfaces. These should conform to the shape of the muscles of the cheek and tongue in an effort to utilize their stabilizing power (Fig. 9.28).

Easily cleaned contour

This should be considered in conjunction with oral hygiene. Although the appearance is unnatural, a smooth-surfaced contour is given to dentures made for a patient exhibiting poor oral hygiene. Patients with good oral hygiene may be given dentures with the natural tissue accurately reproduced. Such patients are given precise instructions for cleaning the dentures to maintain oral hygiene. It should be remembered that good wax-work saves time when finishing the denture and produces a denture which satisfies the patient.

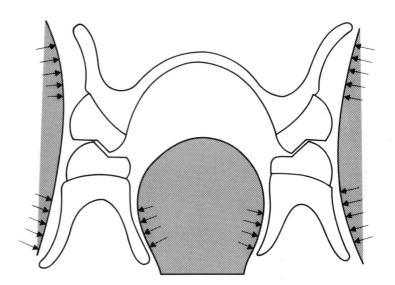

Fig. 9.28 The polished surface of a denture should conform to the shape of the cheeks and tongue.

1 The wax is melted around the necks of teeth to secure them firmly, and all roughened areas are smoothed by use of a hot wax knife.

2 Wax is added around the necks of the teeth to form a gingival roll. This is accomplished by using a wax knife or wax carver in the manner of a pen. Wax is picked up on the tip of the blade, and the handle end of the blade heated to ensure that the wax flows towards the tip of the blade. The edge of the globule of wax is placed against the appropriate area, and the shape of the roll drawn by trailing the globule of wax around the necks of the teeth. The same method is used to form the shape of roots of teeth. Finally, any superfluous depressions are filled in the same manner.

3 The wax is cooled by quenching in cold water. As wax cools, it contracts and may cause slight movement of the teeth. It is advisable to reassemble the denture on the articulator at this stage, to check the occlusion and articulation. Discrepancies are corrected by inserting a warm wax knife at the neck of the appropriate teeth and twisting the blade. Holes caused by the action of the knife are filled with wax.

4 The gingival wax is trimmed, a Le Cron or Ash No. 5 wax carver being ideal for this purpose. The instrument is held in the manner of a pen, with the tip of the blade placed at the centre of the cervical margin of the tooth and the body of the instrument almost contacting the side of the cast (Fig. 9.29). The cast is held in the other hand with the index finger on the occlusal surface or incisal edge of a tooth, whilst the tip of the thumb rests against the cast opposite the tooth around which the wax is to be carved. The hand holding the instrument is supported by its fourth finger resting on the cast, with the body of the instrument trapped between the middle finger of this hand and the thumb of the other hand. The blade is kept at 90° or more to the cervical margin of the tooth and rotated between finger and thumb whilst pressure from the thumb moves the instrument to the right. Pressure from the middle finger of the other hand moves the instrument to the left to complete the cervical contour.

Realistic effects can be achieved by allowing the wax to cover parts of some teeth whilst exposing maximum tooth area on others (Fig. 9.27). All traces of wax must be removed from exposed areas

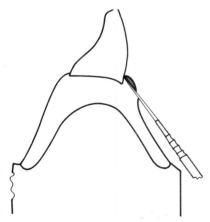

Fig. 9.29 The gingiva is trimmed by use of a Le Cron carver.

of teeth. The hand is supported by the fourth finger resting on the occlusal surface of the teeth whilst the instrument traverses and strokes the surface of the tooth.

When trimming the palatal or lingual gingival contour the angle of the carver is restricted by the palatal or lingual plaster of the cast. This may result in the formation of a ledge around the necks of teeth, especially in the interstitial areas. This ledge is removed by supporting the hand on the occlusal surface of the teeth and carving the wax. The cingulum is exposed on anterior teeth, and the wax given a natural contour without the formation of a plateau.

5 Contouring. The cast is held in one hand, the back of which is rested on a bench peg so that the muscles of the arms are relaxed and the movements of the hands controlled. A wax carver is held in the manner described for gingival contouring but only about 1·5 mm of the blade exposed from between the fingers. A slight twist of the wrist is used to rotate the instrument around the tip of the thumb to shape the wax. Holes in the wax, due to the presence of trapped air, are filled with molten wax.

6 Smoothing the wax. Every effort is made throughout to keep the wax smooth, but final smoothing is accomplished by flaming. This entails brushing a fine flame quickly over the wax to melt its surface momentarily. Excessive heat will cause the wax to run and destroy the contours. A Bunsen burner flame of the microburner type is ideal and mouth blowpipes are also available. The flame must be kept away from acrylic resin teeth, which scorch easily. Where these teeth are used, the denture is held with the teeth facing the burner and the flame brushed quickly over the surface of the wax, which takes on a sheen. Air holes which appear in the wax are filled, the surface smoothed and then reflamed.

7 Polishing the wax. The smoothed wax denture is placed in cold water to harden, then rubbed with wet cotton wool. This produces a high polish. Water left on the surface of the wax is blown off by compressed air to maintain the high gloss; it may be wiped off with cotton wool, but this tends to decrease the gloss.

8 Stippling. This is best attempted after polishing the wax, since vigorous rubbing can destroy the stippling. A toothbrush is ideal for producing this effect if the bristles are reduced to about 5 mm length. The bristles are jabbed into the surface of the wax to produce tiny holes. A pleasing effect can be obtained by stippling in this manner and then flaming the wax to destroy much of the stippling, thereby leaving only odd pockets. Some operators prefer to stipple the acrylic resin denture base during its finishing stage.

9 Finally, the casts are cleaned of wax. The waxed dentures are removed and the casts soaked in water before removing the wax by pouring boiling water over them. Failure to soak the casts causes the mounting plaster to fracture from the casts. All plaster-work is dried and cleaned by rubbing with sandpaper.

10 It is advisable to recheck the occlusion and articulation before presenting the dentures to the surgery.

Waxing partial dentures

The principles outlined for waxing full dentures apply equally to waxing partial dentures. There are just a few areas which require special mention.

Gingival contour. A regular gingival roll should be avoided because the patient can compare the denture with the natural dentition. The gingival contour, therefore, is shaped to harmonize with the natural tissue present (Fig. 9.30).

The peripheral outline of the flanges should be such that they are inconspicuous in the mouth. This is accomplished by terminating a flange in a depression between the roots of teeth and tapering it to blend into the tissues (Fig. 9.30).

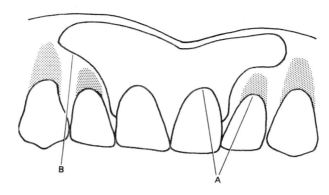

Fig. 9.30 A, the gingival contour of partial dentures is harmonized with the natural tissue present; B, flanges should be inconspicuous by terminating in a depresssion between the roots of teeth.

10 Flask, Pack and Finish Procedures

It is normal to try a wax denture in the patient's mouth, to allow the surgeon to check the jaw relationship recorded earlier, and to give the patient an opportunity to approve the appearance. If alterations are considered necessary, minor adjustments may be made at the chairside, but major changes are carried out in the laboratory, and the dentures are retried in the patient's mouth at a later visit. After the denture has been approved by the patient and surgeon, its base is converted into a hard material. The material most generally used is polymethyl-methacrylate. The conversion procedure is another form of the lost wax process, in that the denture is covered in an investing medium, the wax removed and the resultant mould filled with denture base material.

PREPARATION OF THE WAX BASE

The following stages are carried out on a duplicate cast. It may be necessary to remove the palate of an upper wax base if the duplicate cast contains relieved areas, because these will prevent the denture seating correctly. The wax base is carefully sealed with wax to the periphery of the cast. Failure to do so may result in plaster seeping on to the fitting surface of the cast during subsequent stages.

FLASKS

The denture is embedded in plaster of Paris which is confined within a metal container called a flask. There are many types of flask but basically they consist of two sections each with either a removable base or a large hole with a metal covering disc. Sometimes one section may be deeper than the other. Most flasks contain lugs on one section with a housing for locating the lugs on the opposing section.

Flasking full dentures

1 The flask is checked for cleanliness and to ensure the sections fit closely. The inside of each section is then lubricated lightly with petroleum jelly.

2 The base of the cast is trimmed to produce an inward taper (Fig. 10.1). It may be necessary also to reduce its thickness to ensure that the denture will fit inside the flask. The cast is soaked in cold water for about 10 minutes.

3 A plaster–water mix is made and poured into the shallow section of the flask until about 3 mm from the rim, the cast will displace plaster and raise it to the rim of the flask. The cast is seated into the plaster, keeping the following points in mind.

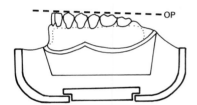

a Where possible, the periphery of the wax should be level with the rim of the flask (Fig. 10.1).

b Where possible the occlusal surface of the teeth should be parallel to the rim of the flask (Fig. 10.1).

c The cast should be tilted to eliminate alveolar undercuts. This is especially necessary when anterior undercuts are present (Fig. 10.1). However, the tilting must not produce a further undercut lingual to anterior teeth (Fig. 10.1), which would prevent the flask being opened without damaging the acrylic resin denture base.

d Plaster should be taken to the necks of gum-fitted teeth (Fig. 10.2).

e The retromolar pad and tuberosity areas should be protected by plaster (Fig. 10.2).

f The flasking plaster must be devoid of undercuts which would prevent the flask being opened.

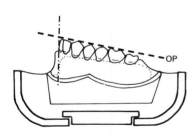

Fig. 10.1 The base of the cast is trimmed to an inward taper and invested with the occlusal plane (OP) parallel to the rim of the flask. The cast is tilted to eliminate an undercut in a cast.

4 The flasking plaster is trimmed whilst it is soft. The flask is held in one hand whilst the blade of a knife is placed on the rim of the

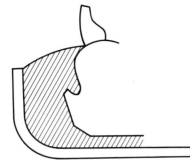

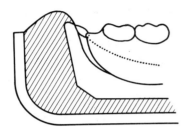

Fig. 10.2 Plaster should be taken to the necks of gum-fitted teeth. The retromolar pad area should be protected by plaster.

flask with its tip fractionally off the wax. It is moved around the flask to remove the excess plaster. The knife is angled to produce a taper on to the posterior border of upper and lower casts.

5 The flask is placed under cold running water as the plaster enters its initial set stage, and the plaster smoothed by gently rubbing a finger over it. Excess water is drained off and the plaster is allowed to set and dry. The rim and lugs should be clear of plaster.

6 A separating medium is applied to the surface of the plaster. Soap solution, waterglass, sodium alginate, oil, wax or petroleum jelly may be used. The last two offer the advantage of producing a slight space between the two layers of plaster which allows space for a thin film of acrylic resin at a later stage. This facility helps to prevent disturbance of the vertical dimension of the denture, which is explained in greater detail later (see packing, p. 171).

7 The opposing section of the flask, minus its base or disc, is assembled over the denture to ensure space exists between the teeth and the top of the flask. The two sections are separated and the disc or base repositioned. It is helpful if the sections of the flask are placed in such a manner as to make assembly easy during the next stage.

8 A further mix of plaster is made and the opposing section of the flask filled to the rim. A little plaster is placed over the waxed denture and vibrated over its surface. The palatal area and lingual aspect of the lowers are completely filled with plaster, the denture inverted on to the opposing section of the flask, which is then closed completely. Excess plaster is removed from the outer surface of the flask, and the flask washed.

9 The initial flasking stage is modified when a metal plate is incorporated as an integral part of a full upper denture base. The first section of the flask is filled with plaster and the denture inserted into it in the manner previously described. More plaster is placed over the metal plate and smoothed level with the join between wax and metal (Fig. 10.3). This plaster must blend into and become part of the flasking plaster in the posterior region of the denture. This method of flasking prevents:

    a Movement of the metal plate during the packing stage.

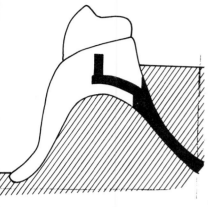

Fig. 10.3 A metal plate should be covered with plaster.

b Acrylic resin covering the plate, which would entail a lengthy finishing technique.

c Scratching or damage to the plate.

Flasking partial dentures

There are two methods available for flasking partial dentures, the open method, which is similar to that described for full dentures, and the hooded method.

Open method

1 The waxed denture, cast and flask are prepared as described for full dentures. The incisal edge and cusps of standing teeth are reduced to wax level to produce a smooth surface, free from undercuts. Care is taken to avoid damaging the proximal surfaces of teeth adjacent to saddle areas.

2 Plaster of Paris is mixed and poured into the deep section of a flask until it is about two-thirds full. The denture is held in both hands with the fingers covering the teeth and flanges, and inserted into the plaster until the teeth are about 1 cm above the rim of the flask. The plaster is taken to the periphery of the wax and all metal components and standing plaster teeth covered with about 5 mm thickness of plaster. The plaster walls should taper to prevent the formation of undercuts (Fig. 10.4), which may occasionally result in part of a wax flange being covered with plaster. The art of good flasking is to produce a mould capable of being opened without fracture of its walls. The surface of the plaster is smoothed and allowed to set completely before coating with a separating medium.

3 A little plaster is placed over the saddle areas of the denture, the flask vibrated to remove air from the plaster, and further plaster added until the saddle areas have been completely filled. The opposing section of the flask is filled with plaster, the denture-holding section inverted on to it and the flask closed. The outside of the flask is cleaned and washed as the plaster reaches its initial set stage.

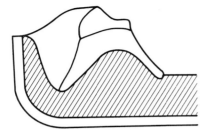

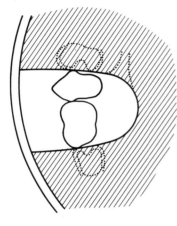

Fig. 10.4 'Open method' of flasking a partial denture. The plaster walls should taper to prevent the formation of undercuts.

Hooded method

The hooded method involves covering the denture teeth with the first mix of flasking plaster and exposing only the palatal or lingual aspect of the denture. As will be seen later this method can be used only when a large space exists between the alveolar ridge and the necks of denture teeth, or when labial or buccal flanges are small or non-existent.

1   The cast and flask are prepared as for the open method of flasking and the deepest section of the flask filled with plaster to within 1 cm of the rim.

2   A small increment of plaster is placed over the labial, buccal and occlusal surfaces of the denture teeth and over wax flanges, and vibrated to eliminate trapped air.

3   The cast is inserted into the flask until at least 1 cm of plaster rises above the occlusal surface of the teeth and the plaster puddled to ensure contact with the labial and buccal aspects of the denture.

4   The plaster is trimmed with a knife to produce an inclined plane from the rim of the flask to the top of the hooding plaster (Fig. 10.5). It is essential that the hood is not reduced below 1 cm in thickness, otherwise it may fracture during subsequent stages.

5   Palatal and lingual metal-work is covered with plaster in the manner described earlier.

6   Topping is carried out in the normal manner.

  This method may also be used when flasking full upper dentures with gum-fitted anterior teeth.

Removing the Wax

1   Operators are reminded that plaster of Paris exhibits an exothermic heat during setting and this can be used to advantage during the next stage, when the wax must be softened before the mould can be opened. If the flask is heated as the exothermic heat develops, sufficient rise in temperature will be produced inside the flask to soften the modelling wax, but not melt it. About 2 litres of

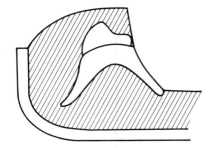

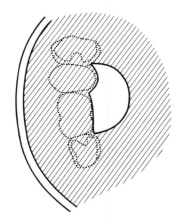

Fig. 10.5 The 'hooded method' of flasking a partial denture. The lingual aspect only is left open.

boiling water is poured over the flask during the initial set stages and the flask left for about 10 minutes.

2   The sections of the flask are prised apart by placing a knife in the appropriate area of the flask. It should be found that the softened wax is capable of being peeled out of the mould. When the open method of flasking is used, the teeth are in one section of the flask and the cast in the other. The hooded method results in the teeth and the cast being in the same section of the flask.

3   The flask is placed on a boiling-out trough, which consists of metal gauze placed over a large container with a syphoning system incorporated. Wax, washed out of the mould, floats on the water in the container. The syphon ensures only water drains away. The wax is removed once it has cooled and hardened. Boiling-out baths are also available from manufacturers.

4   Boiling water is poured over both sections of the mould until every trace of wax has been removed. When, upon opening a flask, the wax is found to be molten, it is possible that the wax will have been absorbed by the walls of the mould. In such cases, detergent is added to the boiling water and the surface of the mould carefully brushed, followed by a further thorough treatment with boiling water. It is often difficult to remove flange wax when the hooded method is used and boiling water must be poured over the mould until it is certain that no wax deposit remains. Sharp edges and loose areas of plaster are removed and the mould rewashed with boiling water. Excess water is allowed to drain off the mould which is left to cool.

PACKING PROCEDURE

The procedure of filling a mould with acrylic resin is termed packing, but before the mould can be packed, the plaster must be treated with a special medium.

Mould preparation

It is essential that the surface of the flasking plaster and cast are coated with a skin-like film. This prevents moisture from the plaster entering and bleaching the acrylic resin. It also prevents monomer from the acrylic resin penetrating the plaster which would cause the plaster to adhere to the denture. Sodium alginate is painted on to all exposed surfaces of the flasking plaster and cast when they are dry and cold. Care is taken to prevent puddles forming around the necks of teeth or to leave a deposit on their undersurface. Excess sodium alginate obliterates the surface details of the mould and may become incorporated in the acrylic resin to produce white streaks. Deposits on the surface of teeth prevents them bonding with the denture base material.

Packing the mould

Methyl-methacrylate resin is produced in two forms, a monomer (liquid) and a polymer (powder). The monomer is very volatile and highly flammable. As monomer changes to a solid state if exposed to light or heat, it must be kept in a tightly sealed, darkened bottle and stored in a cool room. When the monomer and polymer are combined a process called polymerization takes place which produces a hard mass.

1   A glazed pottery vessel, or a polythene container, with a lid is used for the mixing of monomer and polymer. As monomer acts as a solvent, all utensils and the operator's hands must be scrupulously clean. The monomer and polymer are measured by volume in the proportion of 1 part monomer to 3·5 parts of polymer. About 7 cm³ of monomer will be found sufficient for the average full denture; this amount may be adjusted as required according to the size of the denture. The polymer is sprinkled into the monomer, the container being periodically tapped to raise the monomer to the surface so that it 'wets' further additions of polymer. The wet 'sandy' combination formed is mixed thoroughly with a metal spatula, and the lid placed on the container to prevent evaporation of the monomer.

   Various shades of polymer are available, some containing nylon fibres to simulate tissue capillaries (veined). Shades may be produced to harmonize with the patient's tissue by blending the available polymers.

Polymerization of acrylic resin follows a well-defined pattern which is seen as a change in the consistency of the mono-mer–polymer mixture. From the initial wet 'sandy' appearance it becomes stringy and exhibits adhesive properties, this converts to a non-sticky soft dough, which becomes tough, and then hard. The temperature of the vessel in which the acrylic resin is mixed and that of the room in which mixing takes place affects the rate of polymer-ization up to the dough stage. The acrylic resin quickly reaches the dough stage when the mixing vessel and room are hot. The acrylic resin is packed into the mould immediately it reaches the dough stage when it exhibits good flow properties.

2 A metal spatula is used to remove the dough from the mixing vessel. It is formed into a rod, about 15 mm in diameter, carefully placed over the teeth and pressed into the mould with the fingers. About one-third of the dough is flattened and placed over the palatal area of an upper.

The procedure is modified when the hooded method of flask-ing has been used. It takes longer to pack a hooded mould than to pack the open type of mould. For this reason the packing is com-menced whilst still slightly stringy. A small increment of the resin is formed into a roll about 3 mm in diameter and pushed beneath the teeth by the use of a blunt curved instrument. Packing starts at one corner of a saddle so that as the flange fills, the resin will appear at the other end of the saddle. This is continued until sufficient acrylic resin is present to support the teeth. Care is taken not to damage the walls of the mould or to displace teeth. Each saddle is packed in turn, and further increments added to the lingual or palatal aspects of the mould.

3 The two sections of the mould are interlocked and placed cen-trally in a bench press, the handle of which is turned until the top plate of the press contacts the flask and exerts slight pressure to it. The press is given a further turn after a few minutes. Excess acrylic resin is squeezed out of the mould during the procedure. The flask must be closed completely. Partial closure results in a thick denture base which alters the vertical dimension. Too much pressure during closure causes the teeth to compress the flasking plaster and also increases the vertical dimension. Since it is impossible to squeeze all the excess acrylic resin (the flash) from between the surfaces of the flasking plaster, some slight alteration to the vertical dimension is inevitable unless provision is made for it during the flasking procedure. Space may be provided for the flash by using wax or petroleum jelly as a separating medium during the flasking procedure.

4   It is possible to open the flask during the closure stage and remove the flash or make additions. The above procedure is modified when a trial closure is used.

> **a**   The tooth-holding section of the mould only is coated with separating medium.
> **b**   Acrylic resin is packed into the coated mould in the manner described.
> **c**   A sheet of Cellophane or polythene is placed over the acrylic resin, the flask assembled and submitted to pressure as described.
> **d**   The application of pressure is stopped with the flask about 2 mm open. The flask is opened, the polythene removed and the flash removed leaving about 2 mm around the walls of the mould. Additions of acrylic resin are made at this stage.
> **e**   The unsealed section of the mould is coated with sodium alginate which is allowed to dry.
> **f**   The flask is reassembled and submitted to pressure until the metal rims of the flask contact.

5   The flask is removed from the bench press and immediately placed in a spring-loaded hand press ready for the polymerization process. Lack of pressure during this process results in minute voids forming in the acrylic resin called porosity. This is due to the acrylic resin contracting during the polymerization process resulting in contraction porosity.

Polymerization process

The process of converting the acrylic resin dough into a hard mass is accomplished by raising the temperature of the mould. It is called curing, processing or polymerization. The term polymerization is to be preferred because it describes the process taking place, i.e. one of converting the monomer into a polymer. Polymerization is accompanied by an exothermic rise in temperature which may vaporize the monomer when it reaches 100·3°C. This produces gaseous porosity which appears as voids in the thick areas of the denture base nearest the centre of the flask. It is essential that the external temperature of the flask, combined with the internal exothermic rise in temperature never exceeds 100°C when free monomer is present during the early stages of polymerization.

1   The flask is placed in a water bath, the temperature of the water being 20–30°C (a dry heat oven may be used as an alternative.) The temperature of the water is raised to 60°C over a period of 30 minutes and held at that temperature for 30 minutes, allowing the temperature to become evenly distributed throughout the flask.

2   The temperature of the water is raised to 70°C over a period of 30 minutes and held there for 30 minutes.

3   The temperature is now raised to 80°C over a 30-minute period and held there for 30 minutes.

4   Finally, the water temperature is raised to 100°C and held there for 1 hour. This is said to be essential for maximum polymerization and for improving the physical properties of the acrylic resin.

5   The flask is removed from the water bath and allowed to cool to room temperature before progressing to the next stage.

Electrically controlled water baths and dry heat ovens are available, most being fitted with time switches and thermostats which automatically control the temperature rise. A long, slow polymerization process of about 8 hours is to be recommended to minimize the risk of gaseous porosity and to encourage complete polymerization of the acrylic resin.

Pour technique

This method consists of mixing an autopolymerizing acrylic resin to a liquid consistency and pouring it into a mould. The flasking

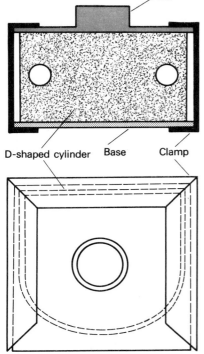

Lid

D-shaped cylinder   Base   Clamp

Fig. 10.6 Type of flask used in the pour technique.

procedure is modified to utilize a reversible hydrocolloid as the embedding medium instead of plaster of Paris, since autopolymerizing acrylic is chemically activated and does not require the application of external heat.

1 The flask used consists of a square metal base, a D-shaped cylinder with two large holes in its flat portion, a square metal lid with a hollow circular extension, a U-shaped box-clamp containing two holes in its rear section, and two cone-shaped bungs for placing in the holes in the rear of the flask (Fig. 10.6).

2 The denture is sealed to the duplicate cast which is trimmed with a slight outwards taper (Fig. 10.7) and soaked in water for at least 10 minutes.

3 The cast is placed on the base plate. The flask is assembled around the denture with the posterior border of the denture facing the posterior holes in the flask, and the holes filled with the bungs.

4 A reversible hydrocolloid is heated as described in Chapter 2, and cooled to 50°C. It is poured into the flask through the hole in the lid until it reaches the rim. It is allowed to gel.

5 The flask is taken apart and the cast and denture removed from the colloid mould. The teeth are removed from the wax denture, placed in a gauze tray and the wax removed from the teeth with boiling water. The wax denture base is peeled off the cast and traces of wax removed by pouring boiling water over the cast.

6 The bungs are removed from the embedding medium and two holes cut into the mould to the posterior region of the denture. The holes should be about 10 mm in diameter tapering to about 3 mm diameter at the border of the denture.

7 The teeth are reassembled in the mould. The cast is coated with sodium alginate, repositioned in the mould and the flask reassembled.

8 Autopolymerizing acrylic resin is mixed to a fluid consistency and poured into the mould through one of the posterior holes; the second hole acts as an air vent. Pouring is stopped when acrylic resin rises up the second hole (Fig. 10.7).

9 The flask is placed in a pressure chamber under a pressure of 105 kN/m² (15 psi) for 30–40 minutes.

10 Deflasking consists of removing the colloidal embedding

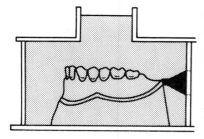

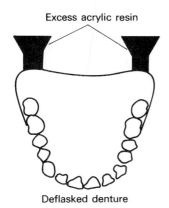

Excess acrylic resin

Deflasked denture

Fig. 10.7 The cast is trimmed to an outward taper and funnels and sprue holes cut into the duplicating material.

material from the denture and cast. Removal of the cast from the denture is accomplished in the manner described for heat-polymerized acrylic resins. The hydrocolloid is washed and placed in an airtight sealable container ready for reuse.

DEFLASKING PROCEDURE

The procedure of removing a denture from its embedding plaster is termed deflasking. This should be carried out carefully to prevent breakage of teeth or the denture base. The spring clamp is released and the flask removed. The embedding plaster is removed from the flask by tapping the centre discs with a wooden mallet. The flask is cleaned ready for further use.

Deflasking full dentures

1   The denture is deflasked by making six saw cuts an equal distance apart and about 10 mm deep, around the embedding plaster block surrounding the cast. A knife is inserted into one cut and twisted to break the plaster (Fig. 10.8). This is repeated in all the saw cuts until the final segment remains, which is removed by placing the knife between the exposed cast and the segment of plaster and twisting to break it away from the cast.
2   The acrylic resin flash is fractured off. Failure to do so may result in cut fingers.
3   The cast is removed by making a series of saw cuts at an angle to the posterior border of the denture commencing near the tuberosity or retromolar pad and prising each section off (Fig. 10.8). Care is taken not to cut the denture or fracture it. It is advisable to chip the cast away when an undercut exists. A half-round sculptor is used in the manner shown in Fig. 1.4 (see p. 8). It may also be necessary to chip the final anterior section of the cast out of the denture.
4   Finally, saw cuts are made in the remaining investing plaster. The first cut is made in the area of the centrals, a further two in the region of the last molar on each side of the denture. Knife pressure

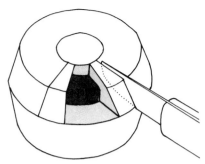

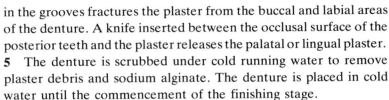

in the grooves fractures the plaster from the buccal and labial areas of the denture. A knife inserted between the occlusal surface of the posterior teeth and the plaster releases the palatal or lingual plaster.

5 The denture is scrubbed under cold running water to remove plaster debris and sodium alginate. The denture is placed in cold water until the commencement of the finishing stage.

Deflasking partial dentures

Partial dentures are deflasked in a manner similar to deflasking full dentures. Greater care is required so as not to damage a metal substructure or to fracture an acrylic resin base, which may require greater use of the sculptor. Deflasking of hooded dentures is commenced by placing a knife blade between the two sections of investing plaster and prising them apart. The topping plaster should be easily removed, coming away with the top section of the flask. The buccal and labial plaster is next removed as previously described, followed by that covering the occlusal, palatal or lingual aspects. The cast is the final section to be removed; it is chiselled away from clasps, followed by removing it in the manner described for full dentures.

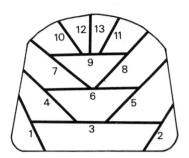

Fig. 10.8 Stages of deflasking a denture. Numerous saw cuts are made in the base of the cast and each section prised off the denture.

FINISHING PROCEDURE

The finishing of a denture consists of two procedures, 1, shaping and smoothing, followed by, 2, polishing. A smooth wax pattern correctly flasked produces a denture requiring little smoothing besides removing the flash.

Shaping

1 Rotary abrasive wheels and points are available for the shaping of dentures. Their effectiveness depends upon: the hardness of the abrasive; the shape and size of the abrasive particles; the rate of movement of the rotary instrument; and the pressure applied. The selection of such instruments is large. The most efficient are those which remove material quickly yet leave the surface of the denture smooth.

The flash is removed by use of a 7·5 cm (3 inch) carborundum wheel attached to the spindle of a dental lathe. The motor must rotate towards the operator in an anticlockwise direction and be within the confines of a rubber trough (see p. 16, Fig. 1.10) which offers protection to the operator. The grinding wheel may be thought of as consisting of twelve sections like a clock-face. The denture is held in both hands with the teeth facing downwards and is pressed against the wheel in the 7–8 o'clock region (see p. 16, Fig. 1.10). The flash only is removed, care being taken not to grind the periphery of the denture.

2   Surface roughness is smoothed by small rotary stones secured in a handpiece. The handpiece is held with the thumb resting on the denture and the grinding stone lightly brushed over the surface of the denture. Rough areas only of the denture base are ground. The posterior border of an upper denture is shaped to the edge of the peripheral post dam and given a gradual chamfer.

3   Ground areas are further smoothed by rubbing with fine sandpaper. The smoother the denture base, the quicker and easier it is to polish.

4   The fitting surface of the denture is scrutinized for irregularities, any present being removed by use of a half-round sculptor.

5   Small rotary points or burs are used to remove the flash from around the saddles of partial dentures. Care being taken not to damage contact areas. It can be helpful to outline the contact area on the denture in pencil lead and to make sure it is not removed until grinding is complete.

6   All dentures should be seated on the master cast to check the accuracy of fit. Selective grinding may be necessary to obtain an accurate fit.

7   Pieces of plaster of Paris adhering between teeth are removed by use of a pointed instrument. Irregularities around teeth, caused by air inclusion in the mould, are removed by use of a flat-edged sculptor. Acrylic resin teeth are easily damaged by this instrument.

Areas of plaster of Paris adhering to the denture are removed by soaking in a solution of sodium citrate for 24 hours and then brushing the debris off under running water, or by insertion in an ultrasonic cleaner for 10–15 minutes.

Polishing procedure

Polishing is the term used to describe the final smoothing and shining procedure. It consists of smoothing by use of a mild abrasive (such as pumice) followed by the formation of a highly glossed surface.

1 Pumice is mixed with water to a thin homogeneous consistency in a rubber trough. A partially worn brush (one with about 10 mm length of bristles) is attached to the spindle of a lathe, the lathe set in motion and the brush impregnated with pumice. The denture is held firmly in both hands, with the teeth uppermost and the buccal aspect of the posterior teeth covered with pumice. The gingival and interstitial area is sharply jabbed against the rotating brush which forces the bristles into the interstitial areas to smooth them. The brush is kept moist with pumice throughout. It is the pumice which smooths the denture, a dry brush scorches the acrylic resin and leaves a brown, roughened area. Excessive pressure or a lengthy smoothing procedure around teeth results in acrylic resin teeth losing their surface detail.

2 The shortened brush is exchanged for one with longer bristles. This is kept away from the teeth and the denture moved constantly throughout the procedure to prevent scorching and the formation of brush marks, which are seen as fine streaks.

3 The palate and lingual aspects of the denture are smoothed by use of a brush. A felt cone or palate brush is used for smoothing those areas inaccessible to the long bristle brush.

4 Small, thin, metal-centred brushes are available for smoothing partial dentures.

5 The denture is washed, dried and examined under a strong light for the presence of scratches. Smoothing is repeated if scratches are present.

The denture must be clean before attempting to give it a high gloss. The bristle brush is exchanged for a cloth or lamb's wool mop and the pumice exchanged for a polishing compound or whiting. A lamb's wool mop and whiting gives a smoother finish. A gloss is obtained by creating a rise in temperature on the surface of the denture which causes the surface molecules of the acrylic resin to flow and fill the minute scratches to produce a glossed surface. This microscopically thin layer is called the Bielby layer. Since heat is created during the polishing procedure, it is very easy to scorch the denture base unless it is kept moving. A deep palate is polished by wrapping cotton wool around the spindle of the lathe and pressing the denture against it.

6 Finally, the denture is washed under cold running water and returned to the master cast.

Every effort is made to keep metal components of a partial denture away from the polishing brush to prevent entanglement and consequent distortion of the metal.

QUALITY CONTROL

It is important to recheck the fit, polish and occlusion of dentures before presenting them to the surgery.

Fit

The fitting surface of the denture is checked for blemishes which must be removed and its fit checked on the master cast.

Polish

The polish is examined under a strong light; no scratch marks should be visible.

Occlusion

The occlusion is checked in centric relation, protrusion, and lateral positions. Slight occlusal dysharmony may be noticed by the incisal guidance pin rising off the incisal table. It may also be highlighted by placing a piece of articulating paper between the teeth. Carbon spots are removed by grinding, remembering the BULL rule (see p. 154). Complete harmony is obtained by use of a carborundum paste. The paste (it can be purchased in paste form or formed into a paste in the laboratory by the addition of oil, glycerine or petroleum jelly) is placed on the occlusal surface of the teeth. The articulator is closed and moved to left and right an equal number of times each side, by holding the dentures firmly in contact. Protrusive movements are also exercised. About twenty such movements are made as routine, but they may be increased until balance is re-established.

The dentures are washed and a final occlusal check made. Careless handling of the carborundum paste may necessitate a further polish. The finished dentures should be kept in a medicated solution until required by the dental surgeon. (Dentures contract upon losing water and swell upon regaining. Continual loss and gain of water induces stresses in a denture base which may eventually lead to a fractured or crazed base.)

11 Immediate Dentures

When a full denture is constructed before the extraction of the natural dentition, and fitted into the mouth immediately after extraction of the teeth, it is termed an immediate denture. If the fitting of the same denture is postponed for some hours or days it becomes a postimmediate denture. The alternative is for the patient to remain edentulous until healing is complete and the alveolar bone has stabilized after resorption. This has numerous disadvantages such as, loss of appearance and difficulty in speech, loss of facial contour and muscle tone, difficulty experienced when eating, which may result in temporomandibular joint problems. Immediate dentures can eliminate these disadvantages and offer some advantages. They assist with the formation of blood clots and prevent their disturbance. They prevent food debris entering the sockets and thereby reduce the risk of infection. They prevent a change in the patient's dietary habits which helps to maintain the health of the patient and encourage rapid recovery. Immediate dentures may be of psychological benefit to patients, especially those with public engagements.

PREOPERATIVE PARTIAL DENTURES

Theoretically, it is possible to extract a complete natural dentition and to fit a full denture for a patient whilst the patient is still anaesthetized. Such an experience is traumatic for the patient, and because of the state of the tissues the oral structure is unsuitable for retaining a denture base. Consequently, better stability is obtained if extraction and replacement is introduced in two stages. Initially, only the posterior teeth are extracted and a temporary partial denture constructed. This gives time for the alveolar bone to stabil-

181

ize and introduce the patient to dentures. They may be immediate or postimmediate partial dentures. Some time later, the anterior teeth are extracted and a complete denture constructed.

1   Impressions are taken and casts poured. Occlusal rims and bases are constructed where necessary, and the occlusal relationship recorded. Alternatively, a wafer registration may be used. The casts are mounted on an articulator. Posterior teeth are selected from stock with a buccolingual dimension about a third narrower than the natural dentition. This reduces the occlusal forces transmitted to the mucosa. The mesiodistal width should approximate with the natural dentition.

2   A pencil lead line is drawn around the gingival margin of each posterior tooth on one side of the cast only and a piercing saw used to remove the teeth to the line drawn (Fig. 11.1). Each socket is then reduced separately by 2 mm and the gingival plaster trimmed to produce the contour of an edentulous ridge (Fig. 11.1). The process is repeated on the other side of the cast.

3   A wax base is adapted to the cast, but strengtheners are not used because the denture will not be tried in the mouth. A single denture is constructed to articulate with the opposing natural dentition. However, when upper and lower dentures are being constructed, the posterior teeth are set to the compensating curve and balanced occlusion and articulation achieved within the confines dictated by the incisal angle.

4   Additional retention in the form of clasping may be incorpo-

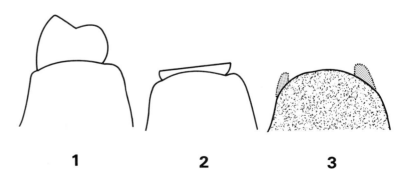

Fig. 11.1   Each tooth is sawn off and the cast trimmed.

1   **2**   **3**

rated in the denture which is then waxed in the manner described in Chapter 9.

5 It is necessary to duplicate the prepared cast. The waxed denture is removed from the cast and placed in cold water. A post dam is carved into the upper cast, and the articulator mounting plaster removed on an electric plaster trimmer. The cast is soaked in water and duplicated in the manner previously described (see Chapter 2).

6 The denture is sealed to the duplicate cast, flasked, packed and finished. The master cast is remounted on the articulator. Normal checking procedures are carried out and the occlusal surface of the teeth spot ground until balance is achieved.

3 The denture is fitted immediately the natural teeth have been extracted. It may be relined (see Chapter 12) as resorption takes place and a full mouth immediate denture constructed when resorption has stabilized.

THE PRESCRIPTION

The prescription for an immediate denture records the normal information required for the construction of dentures, plus information pertaining to surgical procedures and to modifications required to the position of the teeth.

Surgical information

This includes such details as:
1 The type of operation to be performed, a simple extraction or reshaping of the alveolar process by septal alveolectomy.
2 The depth of the gingival crevice.
3 The compressibility of the oral tissues.
4 The depth of the socket to be cut into the cast.

Tooth information

This includes information regarding modifications to the incisal length, anteroposterior position of anterior teeth, their shape and arrangement. Also included is the form the denture base is to take, whether it is to have a complete labial flange or contain a labial gum slip, be partially flanged, or open-faced.

CONSTRUCTION OF INDIVIDUAL TEETH

Immediate dentures can be constructed using stock denture teeth or individual teeth may be produced to the patient's requirements. The construction of individual teeth requires a replica of the teeth from which to make a mould. The replicas (pattern) may be formed in wax, soluble plaster, plaster of Paris or dental stone.

1 An irreversible hydrocolloid impression of the patient's mouth may be used or a duplicate impression may be taken from the master cast.

2 Modelling wax is melted in a small ladle. When almost cool, but still fluid, it is poured into the mould in one continuous stream until about 3 mm above the gingival margins of the teeth. Two pieces of bent wire may be inserted into the setting wax to assist with its removal from the impression. When the wax has set, the impression is placed in cold water to quicken the solidification process.

3 When soluble plaster is used, a mixture of 60% plaster of Paris and 40% starch is added to water and spatulated to a creamy consistency and poured into the impression. This mixture swells and disintegrates when boiling water is poured over it, which is helpful at a later stage.

4 The patterns are removed from the impression en bloc and checked for detail. If detail is not accurate, another cast should be poured.

5 Each tooth is elongated by laying the blade of a wax carver on the face of the tooth and using the tip of the blade to penetrate the gingival crevice to a depth of 2 mm anteriorly and 1·0–1·5 mm palatally, and removing the gingival wax or plaster. The base of each tooth is curved until similar in shape to the crest of the alveolar ridge.

6 The next stage requires a plaster impression of the lingual aspect

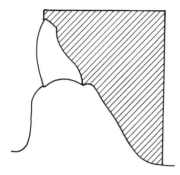

Fig. 11.2 A plaster matrix is formed.

of the standing teeth on the master cast. This area, and about 2 cm of the cast surrounding it, is lubricated with oil or petroleum jelly. A mix of plaster of Paris is made and placed on the prepared area and continued about 2 mm above the incisal edge of the teeth. When the plaster has set, it is released from the cast by pouring boiling water over it. The grease also is removed from the surfaces of the plaster. The plaster block, called a matrix or core, is trimmed (Fig. 11.2). Impression compound may be used as an alternative.

7   The separated teeth are fitted on the matrix. A slight space (diastema) may be observed between each tooth due to loss of material when separating and smoothing. This loss must be made good. Wax is added to the proximal surfaces and the teeth recarved to their original size and shape. Their shape and contact areas are compared to the master cast.

Alternative method

An alternative method is to duplicate the master cast and pour a matrix. The margins of the teeth are outlined with pencil lead, and the teeth removed one by one by use of a piercing saw. The cast is socketed (Fig. 11.3), each socket being about 4 mm deep anteriorly and 1 mm deep palatally, and curved to a typical alveolar ridge shape. The gingival plaster is not removed. The sockets are coated with a separating medium, such as sodium alginate or a soap solution, and the matrix positioned. The central tooth is seated on the

Fig. 11.3 The tooth is sawn off and the cast trimmed.

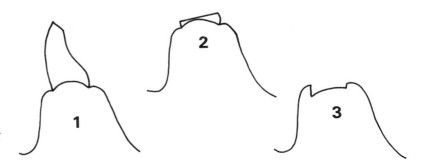

matrix and molten modelling wax dripped into the socket and around the neck of the tooth. The tooth is removed, the wax contoured to shape and then replaced in the matrix. A piece of lubricated tissue paper is placed against the proximal surface of the tooth, the next central positioned and the process repeated. The lubricated paper prevents wax adhering to the previously prepared tooth. All the teeth are positioned in the same manner.

Flasking procedure

The prepared teeth are invested in a small container called a crown flask.

1   Teeth of plaster and soluble plaster are coated with a separating medium, care being taken not to lose surface detail. Wax teeth do not require this treatment.

2   The flask is checked for cleanliness, and to ensure that the sections fit together. The inside is then lubricated. A mix of dental stone is made and the deepest section of the flask filled to the rim. The lingual aspect of the teeth is inserted into the stone, care being taken to prevent air being trapped. The teeth are positioned in a circle with either all the necks or the incisal edges facing the centre of the flask (Fig. 11.4). The labial surface of each tooth should be parallel with the top of the flask, with the stone finishing along the line of maximum convexity of its proximal surface (Fig. 11.4). This is allowed to set and then lubricated. The teeth are covered with a further mix of stone, which is vibrated to eliminate trapped air, the reverse section of the flask filled with the stone and the sections of the flask approximated and closed. The exterior of the flask is washed clean.

3   Once the stone has set, the flask is opened (without preheating) and boiling water poured over both sections. The plaster–starch teeth swell and are eroded by the action of the water, and the wax melts and is washed away. Plaster teeth are removed by inserting the tip of a wax knife under the incisal edge of each tooth and gently prising upwards. A further application of boiling water completes the cleaning of the mould, which is allowed to cool.

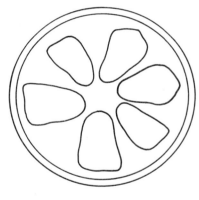

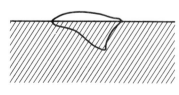

Fig. 11.4   The teeth are positioned in a circle, with the labial surface uppermost.

4   The section of the mould containing the lingual aspect of the teeth is coated with sodium alginate, care being taken to prevent the formation of puddles, and allowed to dry.

Packing procedure

Acrylic resin may be packed into the mould when at the dough stage or the mould may be filled with polymer and the monomer introduced to the mould by use of a pipette. They are termed the dough and powder methods.

Dough method

It will be seen from Fig. 11.5 that teeth consist of two main sections, the body or dentine and the tip or incisal. The dentine constitutes the bulk of the tooth and so is responsible for the shade, the incisal is lighter, often becoming translucent and produces the characteristic lighter incisal edge. Other colours may be added to give the tooth life and vitality.

1   The required shade of dentine and incisal polymer are added to monomer in the proportions of 1 part monomer to 3·5 parts

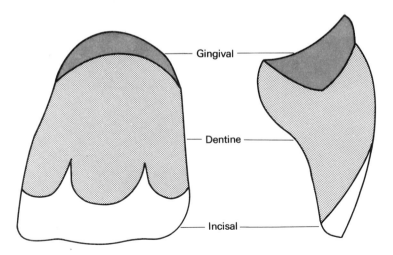

Fig. 11.5   Teeth consist of two main shades and a gingival shade.

polymer each shade being mixed in a separate pot and the mixture allowed to polymerize until the early dough stage is reached. The lingual portion of the mould is filled with the dentine. The flask is covered with a sheet of polythene and then closed under pressure. The flask is removed from the press, opened and excess material cut away.

2   Each tooth is prepared to receive the incisal shade. A portion of the dentine is removed from the labial surface by being chamfered to the incisal edge. The incisal length may be shortened by 1–2 mm and two V-shaped grooves cut into the dentine to form development grooves and introduce translucency (Fig. 11.5). The incisal shade of acrylic resin is placed in the prepared areas, covered with polythene sheet and the flask given a further trial closure.

3   Staining may be added at this stage to produce character and vitality.

Gingival area. The neck or gingival area of a tooth is often darker than the dentine. This is achieved by mixing dentine of a slightly darker shade and placing it in the mould prior to the basic shade of dentine. It should chamfer into the body of the tooth and be covered by the basic shade of dentine (Fig. 11.5).

Enamel crack. This is visible as a broken white line in the natural dentition but it may become stained in time. A razor blade is used to make an oblique cut into the labial surface of the tooth and the acrylic resin raised. The exposed surface is lightly coated with a white stain. Alternatively, a brown stain, nylon thread or a hair may be used to simulate a stained enamel crack (Fig. 11.6).

Decalcification. A sharp instrument is used to cut a small hollow into the surface of the tooth, which is then lightly painted white. This is covered with dentine shade (Fig. 11.6).

Fillings. The introduction of fillings into a tooth, similar to those present in the natural dentition produce a realistic appearance. A half-moon-shaped depression is made at the labioproximal corner of a tooth, the floor of the cavity filled with a darker shade of

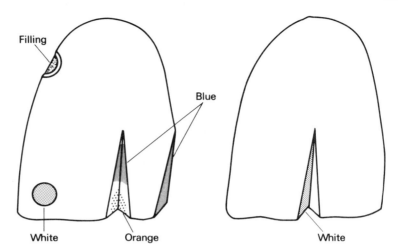

Fig. 11.6 Typical staining which may be incorporated in a tooth.

dentine and then covered with translucent acrylic resin or the original shade of dentine, depending upon the intensity of colour required. The walls of the cavity may be stained brown to simulate an old filling (Fig. 11.6).

Incisal staining. Developmental grooves are cut into the dentine in a V-shape and a trace of orange placed at the incisal edge with blue further along the groove. The stains are covered with dentine, incisal or translucent shade of acrylic resin, depending upon the colour intensity requried.

Surface stains. This is a less effective method of introducing staining but special stains are available which are soluble in methyl-methacrylate monomer.

4   Finally, translucent powder is mixed to a liquid consistency and the surface of the teeth thinly coated with it. The teeth are covered with polythene, the flask assembled, and pressed until the two sections are in metal-to-metal contact. The flask is transferred to a spring-loaded press (many have this combined with the flask).

Ideally, the teeth should be given a lengthy polymerization

process, similar to a denture base material, to produce maximum hardness.

Powder method

1   Both sections of the flasking plaster are coated with sodium alginate which is allowed to dry. The dentine powder is sprinkled into the lingual section of the flask, gingival shade being incorporated when necessary. The dentine is chamfered towards the incisal edge. Monomer is added to the polymer by use of a pipette, and further polymer and monomer added in turn until sufficient is present to fill the mould. It is covered with polythene to prevent evaporation of monomer and allowed to polymerize to the dough stage.

2   The labial surface of the mould is coated with a thin layer of translucent powder, followed by incisal and dentine shades of powder. Staining may be added but it is difficult to control at this stage. Monomer is added by use of a pipette. This is done with care, otherwise the powders will be disturbed and the shade altered. The acrylic resin is covered with polythene until the dough stage of polymerization is reached.

3   The polythene is removed, the flask given a trial closure, opened and staining added. When the flask is full and the tooth has been stained as required, the flask is placed in a spring-loaded press and the acrylic resin polymerized.

Finishing procedure

After polymerization, the teeth are removed from the flask by placing a blade of a knife at the incisal edge of each tooth and prising upwards. Most of the flash can be removed by hand, and the remainder ground away. Care must be taken to prevent damage to the shape and detail of the teeth. They are tried in the plaster matrix and modified until they seat correctly. The teeth are polished on a dental lathe using only whiting and a cloth or wool mop. Care is taken not to polish detail off the labial surface of the teeth.

Cast duplication

When a cast has been socketed during the construction of the teeth and the denture is to be open-faced, the cast is duplicated in the normal manner. The duplicate is mounted on an articulator. This method is used when little or no modification of tooth position is required.

Flanged denture

A labial flange is added to an immediate denture to aid retention. Slight alveolectomy is carried out at the time of extraction of the natural dentition to produce a smooth rounded contour to the gingival area of the tissue. The alveolectomy allows a flange to be made without distortion to the patient's lip.

1 The teeth are removed from the cast one at a time and the sockets prepared as previously described.

2 The area from the gingival margins to the sulcus of the cast is divided into thirds by drawing lines on the cast (Fig. 11.7). The

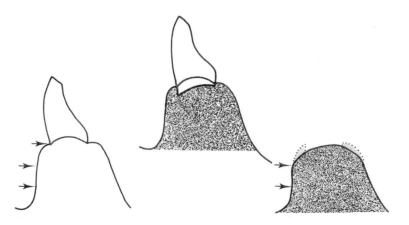

Fig. 11.7 Preparing a cast for a flanged immediate denture. The cast is divided into thirds and the gingival third prepared.

gingival third of plaster is removed to conform to the socket contour already carved (Fig. 11.7).

3 The palatal gingival plaster is removed to form an even contour (Fig. 11.7).

4 The cast is duplicated in the normal manner.

Flanged denture after alveoplasty

Alveoplasty is the deliberate fracture of the trans-septal bone to cause the outer bone plate to collapse into the socket, thereby reducing the bulkiness of the anterior alveolar bone. The cast is socketed and the labial area divided into thirds as described above. The labial plaster is trimmed to the line drawn nearest to the sulcus area. The bulky gingival two-thirds is reduced to produce a favourable labial contour (Fig. 11.7). The cast is duplicated and the duplicate mounted on an articulator.

Template for alveoplasty

When alveoplasty is to be performed it is helpful for the surgeon to have a clear template to indicate the bone modification required. The template is constructed to the prepared duplicate cast. The cast is coated with soap solution and two layers of modelling wax closely adapted to it. The periphery of the plate is smoothed. The wax is carefully removed from the cast and plaster of Paris poured into it to form a cast. The template is flasked in the manner described for full dentures. It is packed in clear acrylic resin, polymerized and finished. The template is placed in a mild medicated solution until required.

Alternatively, a clear template may be formed from a blank of Perspex which is adapted to the cast under pressure (see p. 16). The template is trimmed and polished in the normal manner.

Setting the teeth

The setting of anterior teeth is carried out by use of the plaster matrix. The sockets are coated with a soap solution and the matrix positioned on the cast. Each tooth is positioned in turn and wax flowed around their necks. When all the anterior teeth have been set the matrix is removed and wax flowed around the lingual aspect. Their positions are modified as required.

The posterior teeth are set on the occlusal rim and base in the manner described in Chapter 9. The denture is then waxed, including a labial flange when required. The anterior teeth may be left as a separate unit from the posteriors, to allow the posterior teeth to be tried in the patient's mouth. This gives the patient an opportunity to view and approve the setting of the anterior teeth. Tooth positions can be modified at the chairside.

Gum slip

The natural colouring of the gingiva may be reproduced in the denture by the use of a gum slip. This is a thin layer of translucent acrylic resin constructed to the contour of the labial wax-work, stained on the inside, and incorporated in the finished denture (Fig. 11.8).

The denture is waxed in the manner previously described. The anterior teeth, premolars, their associated wax-work and cast are lubricated lightly with oil. A mix of plaster of Paris is poured over this area to form a matrix. When set, it is withdrawn from the wax, trimmed, and the oily deposit washed off the plaster with boiling water. A piece of sheet casting wax (0·2–0·4 mm thick) is adapted to the matrix, trimmed neatly to the gingival contour, and sealed to the plaster. The matrix and gum slip are flasked and the mould packed in clear acrylic resin, which is polymerized and finished.

Staining

The inside surface of the gum slip is stained, using soluble acrylic resin stains or Waxeline dyes, applied with an artist's brush. Staining is used to increase or decrease the colour intensity of the denture base material. Tissue colouring is pale where tissue is stretched tight

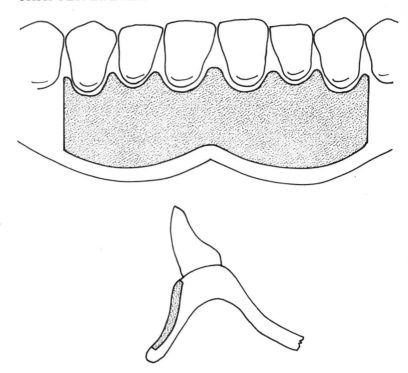

Fig. 11.8 The position and extent of a gum slip.

over the roots of teeth, the depth of colour increasing as the tissue becomes free of bone attachment, e.g. in the sulcus, and where the thickness of the tissue increases, e.g. at the gingival margins of teeth and in the interstitial areas. The required colouring is recorded on a chart, when the tooth shades are taken.

White. This is painted in the root areas. The greatest intensity should be over the canines, less over the centrals and very little over the lateral.

Pink. This is placed interstitially when the denture base material is rather pale. It should be lightly coloured only, to show slight increase in colour intensity.

Pink with blue. The gingival roll has its own characteristic colour, which can vary from a pinky blue, almost mauve, in a healthy mouth, to deep red when gingivitis is present. Pink and blue are mixed on a glass plate and the resultant colour painted on to the gingival roll.

Deep pink. The intensity of pink may be increased to red in the sulcus to simulate loose tissue. Strands of red nylon may also be included to give the appearance of blood capillaries. They are held in position by coating with a clear acrylic resin varnish.

Stabilizing the stain

As most stains are soluble in monomer, it is essential to seal them from the free monomer associated with the packing of a denture. This is achieved by covering the stains with a clear varnish made of clear methyl-methacrylate polymer 15%, chloroform 75% and monomer 10%.

Incorporating the gum slip

There are two ways of incorporating the gum slip in a denture.
1 Wax is removed from the labial surface of the denture, the gum slip positioned and wax recontoured around the slip. The denture is flasked in the normal manner and the wax washed out of the mould. The gum slip should remain in the mould and care taken to prevent its disturbance when packing. The denture is polymerized and finished in the normal manner.
2 The waxed denture is flasked in the normal manner and the wax removed from the mould. The gum slip is inserted into the mould which is packed with acrylic resin. Polymerization and finishing are carried out in the normal manner.

The first method is to be preferred since it is more accurate. The gum slip occasionally proves to be a poor fit against the flasking plaster in the second method which results in the slip being partially embedded in the denture base material.

QUALITY CONTROL

A check of the quality of immediate dentures is essential, especially the fitting surface in the area of the sockets. The gingival area of the teeth must be smooth and polished. The denture is placed in a mild medicated solution until required for surgery.

12 Postfitting Procedures

DUPLICATE DENTURES

A denture may be duplicated as an insurance in case of fracture or because its fit requires improving and yet the patient is pleased with its appearance. The clinician checks the occlusion and vertical dimension. If they are satisfactory, the denture may be duplicated. When they are not satisfactory, the denture is remade commencing with impressions and occlusal rims and bases. For duplication of dentures, a wash impression of zinc oxide–eugenol paste or irreversible hydrocolloid is taken in the denture. The occlusion and vertical dimension are again checked whilst the impression material is setting. Casts are poured in the normal manner. The dentures are removed from the casts, cleaned and returned to the patient. When undercuts are deep, it is necessary to modify the fitting surface of the denture by removal of the denture surface. In this event the procedure is as follows:

1 A cast is poured into the impression.
2 The polished surface of the denture is cleaned.
3 A flask is prepared for use. The shallow section is filled with dental stone and the denture invested in the manner described for waxed dentures.
4 The plaster surface is lubricated. Autopolymerizing silicone rubber is mixed in accordance with the manufacturer's instructions, and applied to the surface of the denture to a thickness of 3–4 mm. This may be covered with metal gauze, to impart strength, the silicone oozing between the mesh. Peripheral extensions of gauze help to retain the silicone in the topping plaster (Fig. 12.1).
5 When the silicone has set, the opposing section of the flask is filled with plaster of Paris and the flasking procedure completed.
6 The silicone allows the flask to be opened, leaving the denture

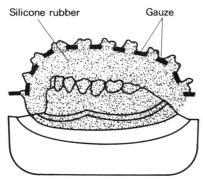

Silicone rubber   Gauze

Fig. 12.1 Duplicating a denture. The silicone rubber oozes between the mesh.

197

attached to the cast, without damage to the mould. The denture is removed from the cast and cleaned. A note is taken of the shade, mould and presence of facets on the teeth. The denture is returned to the patient. Finally, the cast is cleaned of impression material.

7   The next stage is to fit teeth into the mould. Theoretically, it should be possible to place stock teeth in the mould, the necks of the teeth being ground and the flask assembled to check that it will close without interference from the teeth. The task of seating stock teeth becomes difficult if the originals have been ground to obtain balanced articulation. In these instances it is necessary to construct individualized teeth to fit the mould. Two methods are available:

> **a**   Wax is poured into the silicone mould, removed when set, separated into single teeth, and then flasked and packed as described for immediate dentures. These teeth are hard and their appearance can be pleasing, but the technique is a lengthy one.
>
> **b**   The fitting of anterior stock teeth to a mould is reasonably easy, fitting of posteriors is more difficult. Therefore, anterior stock teeth may be used coupled with laboratory-constructed posterior teeth to the shape dictated by the impression. Suitable dentine-coloured autopolymerizing acrylic resin is poured into the posterior portion of the mould until 2 mm above the gingival margins. This section of the flask is placed in a hydroflask under pressure for 10 minutes. The teeth are withdrawn and trimmed until the coronal areas only remain. Damage to the teeth when trimming will result in pink patches on their surface; undertrimming results in dentine-coloured gingival areas. The teeth are left as one unit for each side of the denture. A No. $\frac{1}{2}$ tapered fissure bur is ideal for trimming the interproximal areas. The teeth are replaced in the mould and the flask assembled to check that they do not interfere with its closure. These teeth are of one colour, and soft when compared with heat-polymerized teeth.

8   The exposed flasking plaster is coated with sodium alginate, and denture base material packed into the flask. Overpacking causes pressure within the flask which depresses the silicone to result in a

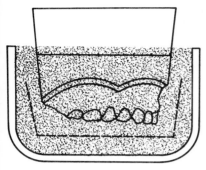

Fig. 12.2 Alternative method of duplicating dentures using an irreversible hydrocolloid impression material.

change in the vertical dimension and imbalance on the occlusal table.

9 The denture is polymerized and finished in the normal manner. Slight occlusal imbalance is corrected at the chairside.

Alternative method

The denture is duplicated in wax, the wax teeth replaced by stock denture teeth, and the denture flasked in the normal manner.

1 An impression is taken in each denture and casts poured in dental stone, or silicone rubber when undercuts are present in the denture. The casts and dentures are mounted on an articulator, the vertical dimension recorded, and the plaster trimmed with an outward taper from the periphery of the cast to the top of the mounting plaster (Fig. 12.2). They are soaked in water prior to the next stage.

2 The deeper section of a flask is prepared and filled with irreversible hydrocolloid. Impression material is pressed into the interstitial areas between the teeth of the denture and the denture and cast inserted into the flask (Fig. 12.2). When the impression material sets, the denture and cast are removed from the flask.

3 The impression is removed from the flask and two tapering holes cut through the material, one at each retromolar pad or tuberosity region. They should commence at a diameter of 10 mm on the outside of the mould and taper to 3 mm on the inside. The denture is removed from the cast and the cast coated with sodium alginate. The cast is returned to the mould and molten modelling wax poured down one hole only, until wax appears at the other hole. The wax is allowed to harden, and the mould is then destroyed to release the wax denture. The dentures can now be returned to the patient.

4 When the results are considered satisfactory, a further impression is taken of the denture in irreversible hydrocolloid and a stone cast produced for checking the appearance of the duplicate dentures.

5 The cast is returned to the articulator with the wax dentures *in situ*. Teeth of the required shade and mould are selected. One wax tooth is sawn off and a stock denture tooth positioned in its place without damage to the gingival wax-work. This is repeated for each tooth until all occlude with the opposing wax teeth. The lowers are set to the upper teeth. The dentures are checked for balanced articulation and may be tried in the mouth.

6 The cast may be duplicated and the denture flasked on the duplicate. After finishing procedures have been carried out, the denture is returned to the master cast and articulation checked and modified if necessary. The finished denture is ready for insertion into the patient's mouth (see Appendix for recent developments by R. Yemm *et al.*).

RELINING

The alveolar bone undergoes changes after extraction of the natural dentition. After an immediate denture has been fitted these changes eventually result in a deterioration of the fit. The fitting surface of the denture requires occasional modification if a reasonable fit is to be maintained. This is achieved by 'relining', that is lining the fitting surface of the denture with a layer of acrylic resin. An impression of the changed surface of the alveolar tissues is necessary. Zinc oxide–eugenol paste or an impression wax is used inside the denture, care being taken not to disturb the occlusal relationship nor to increase the vertical dimension. It may be necessary to remove undercut areas from the fitting surface of the denture and to modify the periphery before taking an impression.

1 The polished surface of the denture is cleaned of impression material, with the exception of its periphery, and a cast poured.

2 A flask is prepared for use and the denture invested in the manner described for a wax denture.

3 The flask is opened and wax impression material completely removed by use of boiling water. Zinc oxide-eugenol paste is gently scraped or peeled off, not washed, portions of the material adhering to the denture being removed by use of a solvent such as Krex, which is also used to clean the fitting surface of the denture. Thorough cleaning is essential because eugenol reacts with acrylic resin to retard its polymerization process.

4 All exposed plaster areas are coated with sodium alginate, care being taken not to coat the denture surface, especially in the peripheral area, because sodium alginate produces a white demarcation line between new and old acrylic resin.

5 The acrylic resin is mixed as described in Chapter 10, and allowed to polymerize to the dough stage. The fitting surface of the denture is moistened sparingly with monomer and the mould packed with the dough.

6 Rapid polymerization is necessary to prevent warpage of the previously polymerized base. The flask is placed in cold water, which is brought to the boil in 30 minutes, followed by boiling for 30 minutes. Alternatively, autopolymerizing acrylic resin may be used.

7 The polymerized denture is deflasked in the manner previously described. Its periphery is smoothed and the denture polished.

Care should be taken throughout the procedure to prevent an increase in the vertical dimension.

REBASING

Rebasing is the construction of a complete new denture base without altering the position of the teeth and without using new teeth. This method is used when alveolar bone changes are excessive, when a denture has been repaired many times, or as a method of repair when the denture has been fractured into many pieces. When the denture is complete an impression is taken in the denture; when the denture is fractured, an impression is taken of the mouth in a stock tray.

1 A cast is poured into the impression.

2 The polished surface of the denture is cleaned.

3 The denture and cast are flasked in the shallow section of a flask.

4 Flasking is completed using silicone rubber covered with plaster of Paris in the manner described for duplicating dentures (see p. 197).

5 When the investing materials have set, the denture is removed from the flask and the denture and cast cleaned of impression material. Denture base material is removed with a grinding wheel until only the teeth remain on a 5 mm wide section of the base directly over the crest of the alveolar ridge (Fig. 12.3), resembling

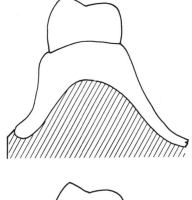
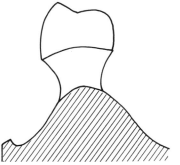

Fig. 12.3 Rebasing a denture requires most of the denture base material being removed, except for a thin area beneath the teeth.

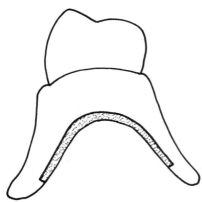

the shape of a horseshoe. Denture base material present around and between teeth is removed with No. 3 and No. ½ flat fissure burs, so that the rebasing material will terminate at the neck of each tooth (Fig. 12.3). The remaining denture base material is thoroughly cleaned under running water.

6   A post dam is cut into an upper cast. The teeth are firmly seated into the flask and the denture constructed in the normal way.

RESILIENT LINERS

The fitting surface of a denture may be lined with a flexible material referred to as a soft or resilient liner, when a denture base pressurizes a bony prominence or when an elderly patient suffers from an excessive resorption of the lower alveolar ridge. The liner may be inserted during the construction of the denture or after its construction. The latter method allows the denture to be finished and tried in the mouth, so that the occlusion and articulation may be checked before the addition of the resilient liner. The introduction of a resilient liner during the construction of a denture base allows the use of a heat polymerized silicone rubber.

1   The denture is constructed in wax, tried in the patient's mouth, and any necessary adjustment made.

2   The denture is removed from the cast and a spacer formed in shellac or wax to a thickness of 2 mm. The spacer is either adapted to the whole of the fitting surface of the cast or to terminate short of the sulcus (Fig. 12.4), the second method being preferable because the periphery of a denture protects the liner from being accidentally torn off the denture base during use. The liner is removed from the cast and placed in cold water until required.

3   The denture is sealed to the cast and flasked in the normal manner. After removal of the wax, the mould is coated with sodium alginate, the spacer placed on the cast and the spacer and cast covered with polythene to separate them from the acrylic resin. The flask is filled with acrylic resin and given a trial closure. Upon opening the flask, the excess acrylic resin is removed, the flask reclosed and polymerization continued at room temperature for 30 minutes, with the flask under pressure.

Fig. 12.4   A resilient liner may cover the whole of the fitting surface of a denture or it may terminate short of the sulcus.

4   The flask is opened, the spacer removed and the plaster re-coated with sodium alginate.

5   The silicone is squeezed from a tube directly on to the surface of the denture base (polymerization commences immediately the material becomes exposed to the air). The flask is closed under pressure and clamped.

6   The denture is polymerized in the normal manner. Deflasking is carried out with great care. The bond between liner and denture base can be broken by careless handling.

Alternative method

The denture is finished in the normal manner, tried in the patient's mouth and occlusal adjustments completed.

1   The denture is returned to the master cast and a matrix formed to the occlusal and lingual surface of the denture. These are mounted on an articulator and the vertical dimension recorded.

2   The denture is removed from the cast and a minimum of 2 mm of the base material cut from the fitting surface, preferably finishing short of the periphery of the denture (Fig. 12.4). The denture base is cleaned under cold running water.

3   The fitting surface of the denture is coated with a silicone adhesive (supplied by the manufacturer) which is dried carefully by holding the denture well above a Bunsen burner flame until a white bloom is developed. The bond between the denture base and resilient liner, will be impaired if the prepared surface is touched by hand.

4   The cast is coated with sodium alginate. The silicone paste is squeezed from its tube on to a pad, an accelerator added and the two mixed thoroughly. The paste is added to the surface of the denture with a spatula, and the articulator closed.

5   Polymerization takes about 15 minutes, depending upon the amount of accelerator used.

Finishing procedure

Resilient liners are difficult to trim and polish. Flash at the periphery of a denture is firstly trimmed by use of scissors, followed by a rotating abrasive trimmer. It is important to trim from liner to denture base, to prevent the liner being torn off the base. Final smoothing is done by hand with fine sandpaper.

ADDITIONS

After the construction of a partial denture, it occasionally becomes necessary to extract further teeth. These may be replaced by an addition of teeth to the partial denture. The addition may be prepared before extraction for immediate fitting, which is preferable or it can be made immediately after extraction for a postimmediate fitting.

1   The existing partial denture is checked for accuracy of fit in the mouth. Unsatisfactory dentures are remade to include the teeth being extracted. Clasps rendered superfluous because of extraction of teeth are cut off at the point of insertion into the denture base. The surgeon takes an impression over the denture, and the impression with the denture *in situ*, is withdrawn from the mouth and sent to the laboratory.

2   The fitting surface of the denture is lightly lubricated with oil and a cast poured.

3   The denture is removed from the cast. The tooth or teeth to be extracted from the mouth is sawn off the cast, which is prepared in the manner described for an immediate denture (see Chapter 11).

4   The denture is prepared by reducing the height and thickness of the base sufficiently to allow an even contour of the base on to the new tooth or teeth (Fig. 12.5). The edge of the ground area should be rounded and polished with pumice. The denture is replaced on the cast, a stock tooth adapted to the area and its position checked with the opposing cast. It is advisable to articulate casts when more than one tooth is to be added. The tooth is secured with wax and the wax contoured as required.

5   A plaster matrix is formed over the tooth (Fig. 12.5). The wax is removed and the plaster parts coated with sodium alginate.

6   The units are assembled and firmly held in position with elastic

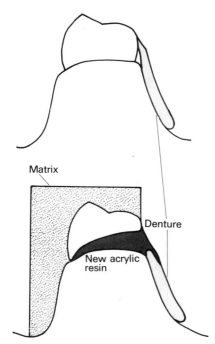

Matrix

Denture

New acrylic resin

Fig. 12.5   Adding a tooth to a partial denture. The surface of the denture is prepared, a denture tooth obtained and a matrix formed.

bands. The prepared area of the denture base is moistened lightly with monomer. Autopolymerizing acrylic resin is mixed to a fluid consistency and poured into the mould until level with the surface of the denture. The assembled units are placed in a hydroflask filled with water at a temperature of 37°C. The lid is positioned and the flask pressurized to a minimum of $140 \, kN/m^2$ (20psi) under a bench press for 15–30 minutes. The use of a hydroflask is essential to minimize the occurrence of porosity in the acrylic resin.

7   After polymerization, the denture is removed from the flask and cast, trimmed to shape and polished. It is placed in a mild antiseptic solution until required.

The addition of a number of teeth, for example the immediate replacement of all the anterior teeth, may be undertaken by flasking in the manner of full dentures using heat-polymerizing acrylic resin.

REPAIRS

When a denture fractures or a tooth breaks off the base, it is advisable to identify the cause of the breakage and if possible prevent its recurrence. The causes fall into three main groups:

1   Intraoral causes. Changes of alveolar bone, denture rocking on a bony prominence producing stresses within the denture base, and a heavy occlusion may eventually cause fracture of the denture base.

2   Incorrect construction techniques. These may include incorrect setting of teeth, inadequate polymerization time, denture base too thin, or a large labial fraenum notch causing a concentration of stresses within the denture base.

3   Accidental mishandling. The patient may drop the denture whilst cleaning it.

If the cause of breakage falls under **1** or **2**, the denture should be modified by relining or should be remade completely.

Fractured lower

Heat- or autopolymerizing acrylic resins may be used to repair a denture. Use of the heat-polymerizing resins require the denture to be flasked and given a long polymerizing period. Although care is necessary to avoid warpage of the base, the repair strength is high. Autopolymerizing acrylic resin eliminates the necessity for both flasking and the lengthy polymerizing process, thus reducing the repair time and eliminating possible warpage of the base, but the repair strength is not as high as that of heat-polymerizing resins.

Using heat-polymerizing resin

1   A check is made to see that the fractured sections interlock before the denture is accepted for repair. The fractured surfaces are approximated, firmly held in position and sealed by dripping model cement (sticky wax) on the polished surface only. The fitting surface is scrutinized to ensure that the pieces are correctly aligned. The joint is strengthened by attaching a piece of wire with sticky wax to the occlusal surface of the teeth on both sides of the denture (Fig. 12.6).

Large undercuts on the fitting surface of the denture may be blocked out by use of wax or plaster of Paris. The plaster is lubricated before pouring a cast.

2   A cast is poured into the denture.

3   The sticky wax is removed and the denture lifted from the cast. The fractured surfaces on the lingual aspect of the denture are trimmed to produce a 2–3 mm space. The edges are rounded (Fig. 12.6). As little as possible is removed from the labial surface so as to ensure that the repair is invisible. Sufficient space must exist between the surfaces to allow acrylic resin to pass from the lingual surface to the labial surface.

4   The prepared surfaces are polished with pumice and thoroughly washed clean. The cast is coated with sodium alginate and the component parts assembled on the cast. The prepared area is filled with wax which is contoured to harmonize with the denture.

5   The base of the cast is trimmed to allow the denture to be flasked using the hooded method. The whole denture, with the exception of about 1 cm either side of the waxed fractured area is embedded in

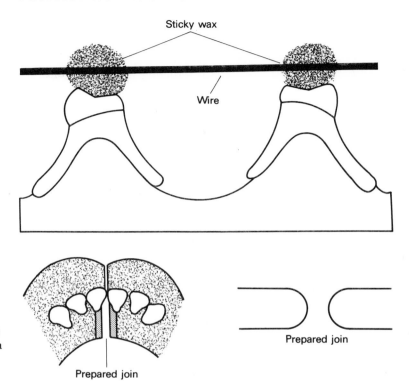

fig. 12.6 The fractured denture is firmly held in position whilst a cast is poured. The joint is prepared as shown.

plaster of Paris (Fig. 12.7). The flasking plaster must be free of undercuts. The flasking procedure is completed.

6 The flask is opened and the wax removed with boiling water. It may be difficult to remove wax from a labial flange and boiling water should be poured into the joint for some time after the wax appears to have been removed.

7 The surface of the joint is dried, and then moistened slightly with monomer. Acrylic resin is mixed to the proportions recommended by the manufacturer and packed into the flask at the dough stage. The dough is formed into a rod about 2 mm in diameter, and forced through the prepared opening on to the labial surface with a thin metal instrument such as the curved end of an Ash No. 5 wax carver. This is followed by filling the lingual aspect to slight excess, closing

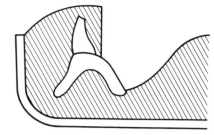

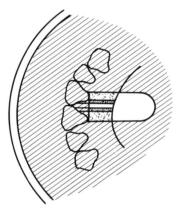

Fig. 12.7 The hooded method of investing is used when repairing a denture by use of heat-polymerizing acrylic resin.

the flask and compressing it in a bench press. It is given a trial closure to ensure sufficient acrylic resin has been packed, and more added if necessary.

8   Polymerization time should be kept to a minimum to prevent distortion of the denture base material. The flask is placed in cold water which is heated to bring it to boiling point in about 30 minutes. It is kept at this temperature for a further 30 minutes, and then removed from the water and allowed to bench cool. The denture is deflasked, the repaired area smoothed and the whole denture polished and cleaned.

Using autopolymerizing resin

1   The component pieces of the denture are assembled and waxed together in the manner previously described and a cast poured.

2   The denture is removed from the cast, the fractured surfaces reduced by about 0·5 mm. The area directly beneath the teeth is ground to produce a space 2 mm wide. The edges of the prepared area rounded and then polished with pumice. The pieces are thoroughly washed clean.

3   The cast is coated with sodium alginate and the components assembled on the cast. Autopolymerizing acrylic resin is mixed to a fluid consistency and dripped into the join to slight excess.

4   The denture, *in situ* on the cast, is placed in a hydroflask with a water temperature of about 37°C and a minimum pressure of 140 kN/m² (20 psi). It is left in the flask for 15–20 minutes. The repaired denture is trimmed and polished in the normal manner.

Fractured upper

Using heat-polymerizing resin

1   The components are assembled and waxed together as previously described and a cast poured.

2   The warpage of a denture base associated with repolymerizing acrylic resin by heat, may be reduced by removal of the whole palate and replacement with new acrylic resin. The palate is removed with a large grinding wheel to within 1 mm of the teeth. The remaining acrylic resin around the teeth is removed with a No. 3 and No. ½ flat fissure bur. The fractured area beneath the teeth is widened to 3 mm tapering to about 0·5 mm at the polished surface of the labial flange.

3   The components are assembled on the cast and the missing portions of the denture recontoured in wax.

4   The denture is flasked using the hooded method, the whole of the palate being exposed but with the teeth completely covered with plaster. Flasking is completed, the wax thoroughly washed off using boiling water and the palate of the cast coated with sodium alginate.

5   The acrylic resin is mixed and packed at the dough stage into the mould. The flask is closed, clamped, and the acrylic resin polymerized in the manner described on p. 172. The denture is deflasked, trimmed and polished in the normal manner.

Using autopolymerizing resin

The fractured sections are waxed together and a cast poured. The line of fracture is prepared in the manner described for a lower denture and the cast coated with sodium alginate. Autopolymerizing acrylic resin is mixed to a fluid consistency and the fracture filled. Polymerization takes place within a hydroflask under pressure. The repaired denture is trimmed and polished.

The strength of an autopolymerizing acrylic resin repair is less than that of a heat-polymerizing resin and may be lower when porosity is present. The advantage of the technique lies in the speed by which the repair can be made and the avoidance of possible distortion of the base which may occur when heat is applied to an existing acrylic resin denture base. Autopolymerizing resins are not recommended for the repair of multiple fractures or when the patient has a heavy occlusion.

Tooth replacement

Teeth may need replacement for several reasons:

    a   Fracture of porcelain teeth due to careless handling.

b Lack of mechanical retention with the denture base allowing teeth to fall off the denture.

c Fracture of acrylic resin teeth due to careless handling.

d Poor technique, i.e. a layer of wax, or sodium alginate on the surface of the teeth at the time of packing, may allow acrylic resin teeth to fall off the denture base.

e Lack of chemical bonding with the denture base may allow acrylic resin teeth to fall off the denture base. Cross-linking agents are included in most acrylic resins to prevent crazing, and increase the strength, but they also reduce the solubility of the acrylic resin by monomer which prevents chemical bonding. This effect is most common when the base has been constructed in an autopolymerizing resin such as the types used during the pour technique of denture construction.

1 If a displaced tooth is available and is undamaged, it is reseated on the denture base and secured with wax. Alternatively, a replacement tooth is obtained and the shape of the denture base modified to accept it. The tooth is held in position with wax which is contoured to the shape of the denture base.

2 A plaster matrix is formed to the labial surface of the tooth and the wax removed by use of boiling water.

3 The undersurface of an acrylic resin tooth is ground and retention holes or grooves cut into it by use of a rose-head bur. The lingual or palatal surface of the denture base is cut to form a box-shape which is the width and depth of the tooth. The denture base should not be thinned to less than 1·5 mm for reasons of strength (Fig. 12.8). The labial gingival roll is left untouched (Fig. 12.8) to make the repair invisible. The prepared area is polished with pumice to prevent a demarcation line between new and old material.

4 The tooth, matrix and denture are assembled, and secured with an elastic band. A fluid mix of autopolymerizing acrylic resin is made and this is dripped into the prepared space. The repair is polymerized in a hydroflask, followed by the normal finishing procedure.

An old denture may craze upon the introduction of a fluid mix

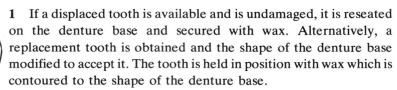

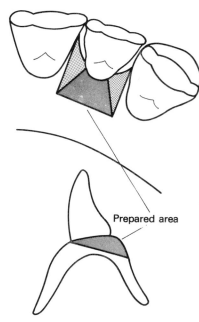

Prepared area

Fig. 12.8 Replacing a tooth. The denture base is prepared, a tooth trimmed to fit the denture and an autopolymerizing acrylic resin used to secure the tooth.

of autopolymerizing acrylic resin, the monomer releasing internal stresses built up in the denture over the years of use. This may be minimized by smearing the adjacent areas of the base with oil or petroleum jelly. It is essential to avoid contamination of the prepared surfaces with the grease, otherwise the chemical bond between new and old acrylic resins will be impaired.

The loss of a number of teeth may necessitate a cast of the opposing dentition to help with articulation. This type of repair is best carried out by using a heat-polymerizing acrylic resin. The denture is prepared as for the autopolymerizing acrylic resin method, but the teeth are secured with wax and no matrix is formed. The denture is flasked on the cast, leaving only the prepared area exposed from the flasking plaster. The wax is removed with boiling water, the denture packed with acrylic resin and polymerized in the manner described on p. 172. Finishing is carried out in the normal manner.

Metal base repair

A fractured metallic denture base is an unusual occurrence, and is usually caused by metal fatigue (possibly due to excessive flexure during function), porosity or foreign inclusions in the metal, or the plate or bar being too thin. It is generally considered best to remake the base to an improved design.

Clasp repair

Fracture of clasps is more common, due partly to metal fatigue and occasionally to distortion from careless handling. Porosity or foreign inclusion may contribute to either of these causes. Repair is accomplished by removal of the fractured unit and replacement with a new wrought or cast component. A new clasp may be embedded and retained in the acrylic resin base constituting the saddle.
1   The surgeon takes an impression over the partial denture. The impression with the denture *in situ*, is forwarded to the laboratory where a cast is poured and a matrix made over the teeth.

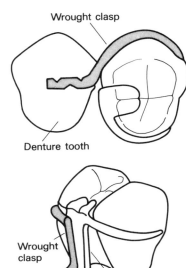

Wrought clasp

Denture tooth

Wrought clasp

Cast unit

Fig. 12.9 Repair of a clasp. The new clasp may be inserted into the saddle of the denture or soldered to another metal unit.

2 The denture is removed from the cast and a wrought clasp adapted to the tooth in the manner described in Chapter 8. The position of the tag is important; it should enter the saddle at the proximal corner of the flange below the teeth (Fig. 12.9). A flat fissure bur is used to cut a groove about 1 cm long into the flange and to penetrate into the centre of the saddle (Fig. 12.9).

3 The tooth being clasped is coated with sodium alginate and the components assembled on the cast. The clasp is secured by use of sticky wax; autopolymerizing acrylic resin is mixed to a fluid consistency and then dripped into the prepared recess. Polymerization is completed in a hydroflask and the denture finished in the normal manner.

Alternative method

An alternative method is to solder the clasp to the metal structure within the saddle area, but the teeth must be removed from the saddle to expose the metal structure. An impression is taken as described above, a cast poured and a matrix constructed.

1 The denture base is removed from the fitting surface of the saddle to expose the metal. This is heated with a microflame, which also softens the denture base. Pressure is applied to the denture base to remove it from the metal. Care is taken to prevent the teeth being scorched.

2 The clasp is constructed with its tag fitting against the metal structure (Fig. 12.9). The surface of the structure and the clasp are cleaned by grinding. The clasp is secured to the cast with a small increment of plaster of Paris over its retentive portion and on to the occlusal surface of the tooth

3 The surfaces to be soldered are fluxed to prevent the formation of oxides. A hydrogen–oxygen generator is used. The flame is directed on to the metal structure adjacent to the tag until the metal becomes a dull red colour. Solder is introduced to the join and immediately it flows, the flame is removed.

4 The soldered area is cleaned by blasting or pickling and the metal polished.

5 Denture base material is removed from the teeth. These are assembled in the matrix and the saddle formed in autopolymerizing acrylic resin. The denture is finished in the normal manner.

It is essential for all the teeth to be removed from a denture base when a town gas–air blow-torch is to be used. The large flame from this type of torch is likely to scorch the acrylic resin attached to the metal structure.

Appendix

Page 9   **Trimming casts.** The procedure given in this book is based upon that described by:

ADAMS C. P. (1975) *The Design and Construction of Removable Orthodontic Appliances.* John Wright, Bristol.

Page 17   **Pressure-formed tray.** The procedure described is based on the Drufomat–U system.

Page 25   **Natural physical forces of retention.**

Adhesion. The attraction that unlike molecules have for each other. It exists between the oral tissues and the saliva, and between the saliva and the denture.

Cohesion. The attraction that like molecules have for each other. It exists within the saliva.

Forces of surface tension. This exists within the saliva around the periphery of a denture.

Atmospheric pressure. This acts on the polished surface of the denture.

Reference:

OSBORNE J. & WILSON H. J. (1974) *Dental Mechanics for Students.* Staples Press, London.

Page 34   **Setting of calcium sulphate.**

Initial set. When the mixture of calcium sulphate and water ceases to be pourable but is sufficiently soft to be carved.

Final set. When the calcium sulphate becomes strong and hard.

214

Page 34   **Humidor.** A chamber used to maintain a constant moisture level (humidity).

Page 45   **Measuring device for occlusal rims.** A measuring device may be formed from a piece of Perspex or a discarded tooth card (Fig. A.1).

Page 116   **Electrolyte for electrolytic polishing of cobalt–chromium alloy.** These may be purchased ready for use or the following solution may be mixed in the laboratory.

Ethylene glycol   80%
Conc. sulphuric acid   15%
Water   5%
The acid is added to the glycol.

Reference:

SHAW F. G. & SCOTT D. C. (1968) *Practical exercises in dental mechanics*. Henry Kimpton, London.

Page 117   **Polishing compound.** Wipla—Weiss Universal—Polierpaste, white or pink polishing compound may be used.

Page 118   **Precipitation hardening.** Details regarding precipitation hardening may be found in:

PHILIPS R. W. (1973) *Skinner's Science of Dental Materials*. W. B. Saunders, Philadelphia.

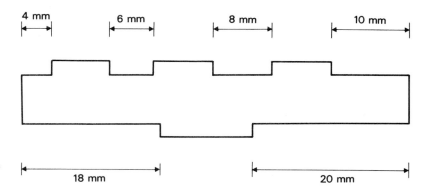

Fig. A.1 A measuring device may be formed to assist with the construction of occlusal rims.

Page 133   **Spot welding.** Further information can be obtained from:

ADAMS C. P. (1975) *The Design and Construction of Removable Orthodontic Appliances*. John Wright, Bristol.

Page 142   **Compensating curves.** In the natural dentition the anteroposterior curve is referred to as the curve of Spee, and the lateral curve as the curve of Monson.

Page 200   **Recent developments in denture copying technique** (Yemm *et al.* *(1978)*.

1   Occlusal relationship is recorded when necessary.

2   An impression of the polished surface of the denture is recorded in silicone putty supported in a disposable tray.

3   The fitting surface of the denture is recorded in silicone putty, supported in a disposable tray. This material must have intimate contact with the first impression.

4   The denture is removed from the impressions and returned to the patient.

5   A shellac base plate is adapted to the silicone impression of the fitting surface of the denture.

6   Pouring holes are cut into the impression of the polished surface of the denture, and the impression assembled to form a mould. Modelling wax is poured into the mould. The impressions, with their trays, are mounted on a plane line articulator.

7   The wax teeth are removed, one at a time; as each wax tooth is removed a denture tooth is attached to the wax plate in its place. The shape of each tooth is modified to fit the impression.

8   The denture is tried in the patient's mouth and a zinc oxide–eugenol paste impression taken of the mouth within the wax denture. The cast is poured and the denture processed in the normal manner.

General Reading List

ADAMS C. P. (1975) *The Design and Construction of Removable Orthodontic Appliances*. John Wright, Bristol.

ANDERSON J. N. & STORER R. (1973) *Immediate and Replacement Dentures*. Blackwell Scientific Publications, Oxford.

BAHRANI A. S., BLAIR G. A. S. & CROSSLAND B. (1965) Slow rate hydraulic forming of stainless steel dentures. *British Dental Journal* **118**, 425.

FENN H. R. B., LIDDELOW K. P. & GIMSON A. P. (1974) *Clinical Dental Prosthetics*. Crosby Lockwood Staples, London.

OSBORNE J. & LAMMIE G. A. (1975) *Partial Dentures*. Blackwell Scientific Publications, Oxford.

PHILIPS R. W. (1973) *Skinner's Science of Dental Materials*. W. B. Saunders, Philadelphia.

SICHER H. & DuBRUL E. L. (1975) *Oral Anatomy*. C. V. Mosby, St Louis.

YEMM R., DUTHIE N., LYON F. F. & STURROCK K. C. (1978) A copying technique for replacement of complete dentures. *British Dental Journal* **144**, 248.

Index

219